Reforming Healthcare

Reforming Healthcare

◆

What the Public Needs to Know

Lindsay Lee Pratt, M.D.

iUniverse, Inc.
New York Lincoln Shanghai

Reforming Healthcare
What the Public Needs to Know

iUniverse, Inc.

For information address:
iUniverse, Inc.
2021 Pine Lake Road, Suite 100
Lincoln, NE 68512
www.iuniverse.com

ISBN: 0-595-29213-5

Printed in the United States of America

Contents

Preface

Have your concerns about the future healthcare delivery system in the United States attracted you to this book? I hope so—you should have those concerns. You may lose the best healthcare delivery system in the world to either another expensive and inefficient government bureauracy or to the investors and business entrepreneurs in the managed healthcare industry. As you read this preface, say to yourself, "Wake up! The healthcare delivery system belongs to me. I receive its services, and I should be in control. Healthcare does not belong to government, to business entrepreneurs, or to investors. Why should they be in control? What do I need to know, and to do, to prevent them from controlling healthcare?" Read this book.

Yes, no other country has been able to provide its citizens quality healthcare services as comprehensively, or as easily available, as those offered by the private delivery system in the United States. However, there are members in Congress as well as businesspersons and investors in the managed healthcare industry (HMOs) seeking legislation to replace the private delivery system with one they can control. Since neither government nor the managed healthcare industry can offer the public a better delivery system, and since they do not possess the training or medical knowledge necessary to improve the services offered by a delivery system, their only interest in controlling healthcare is the power government can obtain and the profits the managed healthcare industry can obtain.

Unfortunately, the public's healthcare concerns have focused on who is going to pay for their services rather than on who is going to be providing those services. Equally important, the public has failed to associate the quality and the availability of their services with the quality and availability of the physicians who provide those services. The public's complacency about healthcare issues has blinded them to the importance of their physicians and to how serious the loss of a private healthcare delivery system would be to themselves and to their families.

This book was written to provide the public the information they need to understand why the private healthcare delivery system is important to themselves and to their families; to understand the existing private healthcare delivery system's problems; and to understand how easily those problems can be resolved by six changes to regulate a private healthcare delivery system.

The materials required to enable the public to become informed healthcare activists are in this book, and using the power of their vote, an informed and politically active public can insure the preservation of a regulated private healthcare delivery system.

In addition, three adenda are discussed. They are:

1. Healthcare Price Controls.

2. Healthcare is not a business.

3. HMOs—Patients Beware!

1

Why this book?

In 1988, while the President of our Medical Society, I began to search for a theme for my presidency. For thirty five years, I had been a busy surgeon/physician, and I had not had the time to think about what was happening to medicine. When I looked at medicine thirty five years later, I did not like what I observed.

The delivery system I had known, called the practice of medicine, no longer existed. I knew medicine as a profession. Its mission was to provide services to all in need of them regardless of their ability to pay. However, the introduction of health and hospital insurance during the 1950s and 60s had transformed the practice of medicine into an insurance driven for-profit business system. Medicine was now called the healthcare delivery system, and its mission was to profit from the delivery of healthcare's services to only those who could afford to purchase them. Furthermore, this insurance driven for-profit delivery system was making it increasingly difficult for those individuals without insurance or without the ability to pay for their services to obtain their necessary healthcare services.

What I saw was an impending problem for my patients and for patients in the future. The government and the managed healthcare industry were using the problems unregulated health and hospital insurance had created for the private healthcare delivery system to advance their agendas to control healthcare. Furthermore, it became obvious to every physician during the 1980s, the government (Medicare) and the managed healthcare industry (HMOs) were becoming less patient and provider friendly as their control of healthcare increased. Their threat to the future healthcare delivery system in the United States had to be brought to the public's attention, and the theme for my Presidency became, "Reforming Heathcare; What the Public Needs to Know."

With both Medicare and the HMO industry becoming less patient and provider friendly, it became obvious the private healthcare delivery system had to be preserved. However, to preserve the private delivery system, a solution had to be found for its escalating costs and for its failure to offer easily available services to those individuals without adequate insurance (Medicaid) or without the ability to pay for their services. To solve healthcare's cost and service availability problems, I proposed six changes to REGULATE the existing private healthcare delivery system.

The six changes were unsuccessfully promoted within the medical community. During the late 1980s and most of the 1990s, insurance companies were not challenging either a physician's services or their fees, and most physicians did not feel threatened by either Medicare or the HMOs. If the six changes were to be adopted, their adoption would require the public's endorsement. It was the public's healthcare delivery system. However, many among the public were not aware of why a private healthcare delivery system was important to themselves or to their families, and they were not aware of the private healthcare delivery system's problems or how easily those problems could be corrected. To provide the public this information, this book was written in 2003, and a search for a publisher was initiated.

2

The Problem, The Cause, The Solution.

The Problem:
The private healthcare delivery system has only two problems. One is the increasing cost of its services, and the other is its failure to provide easily available services to those individuals unable to pay for them. Otherwise, the delivery system has provided the public the most comprehensive, the best quality, and the most easily available services in the world. Furthermore, physicians from all over the world seek the opportunity to obtain training in our private healthcare delivery system.

The Cause:
The only cause of healthcare's two problems has been the introduction of, and subsequent patient and provider abuses of, UNREGULATED health and hospital insurance.

Background:
Employers began offering their employees health and hospital insurance programs during the 1950s and 1960s, and in the mid 1960s, legislation created Medicare and Medicaid. Prior to these insurance programs, the private healthcare delivery system had neither a cost nor a service availability problem, and malpractice litigation was rare. At the time, the patient's pocketbook was the primary source of payment for medical and surgical services. Those patients who could afford to purchase their services questioned their medical necessity, and they purchased only necessary services. Those patients who could not afford to purchase their services were able to obtain free services in outpatient clinics and in inpatient hospital wards.
Based on my experiences as a participating physician and surgeon for more than twenty years in those free clinics and hospital wards, the services offered by those

3

free facilities were of better quality and more easily obtained than most of the services offered by the exisiting insurance driven for-profit healthcare delivery system to Medicaid patients and to patients unable to pay for their services.

During the 1960s, the cost of healthcare's services began to increase. An increasing number of individuals were using health and hospital insurance to obtain their services, and their insurance companies were not monitorng the services their policyholders (patients) were receiving or challenging the increasing provider charges for those services.

Without a challenge from their insurance companies, patients began to demand more and more services and to demand their insurance pay for those additional services. In addition, patients became indifferent to the medical necessity of, as well as the cost of, their healthcare services. Patients were demanding and accepting services more for their convience and desireability than for their medical necessity.

Also, without a challenge from their patients or from their patient's insurance companies, providers began to offer their patients the unnecessary services they were requesting, to charge more for their services, and to charge for services they had been offering without a charge prior to insurance. Furthermore, providers began to unbundle (itemize) their charges. Itemizing enabled them to maximize their insurance reimbursements. In addition, some providers employed lobbyists to acquire legislation mandating insurance programs pay for their services even though some of those services had no medical value.

During the 1960s and 1970s, the increasing patient and provider abuses of health and hospital insurance programs were generating billions of insurance dollars, and as those dollars flowed into the healthcare delivery system, they inflated healthcare's costs from less than 5% of the GNP in 1970 to more than 15% in the 1980s. Those costs, as a percentage of the GNP, are increasing each year. Furthermore, as those billions of insurance dollars flowed into healthcare, they provided healthcare with "deep pockets". Those "deep pockets" attracted attorneys, and the number of frivolous malpractice lawsuits began to increase.

Health and hospital insurance has provided many individuals significant benefits. But what happened to cause something intended to be so good to become so expensive? The answer is the abundance of money offered by unregulated health and hospital insurance.

The following personal experiences offer two example of how insurance money defiled the healthcae delivery system. During the 1950s and most of the 1960s, insurance did not pay for hearing tests, but those tests were available without a charge, or for a minimal charge, in the offices of most physicians who treated ear disorders. In the late 1960s, health insurance began to pay for hearing tests.

The introduction of those insurance payments encouraged many physicians to initiate hearing testing services in their offices, as well as hearing aid sales, even though most of those physicians knew little about hearing testing and even less about hearing aids. Furthermore, the cost of those hearing tests rapidly increased to $100 or more. The second example of how insurance money defiled healthcare occurred in 1975. Responding to a proposal to have Medicare pay for hearing aids as well as hearing tests, I was asked to be the chairman of a Committee to study the hearing aid dispensing system and report to the Food and Drug Administration.

Our committee found existing hearing tests were unable to offer an examiner the information they required to "perscribe" the most appropriate hearing aid for a specific hearing loss. Also, those hearing tests were unable to verify if an individual was wearing an appropriate hearing aid. Accordingly, our report discouraged Medicare payments for hearing aids until more accurate testing procedures were available. The following study explains the reasoning behind our decision.

If the same individual is asked to obtain tests for a hearing aid and for eyeglasses, there is a significant difference in the testing outcomes. When an individual receives five eye examinations from five different examiners, each examiner perscribes eyeglasses with the same lenses. However, when the same individual receives five hearing aid evaluations from five different examiners, the individual receives five different hearing aids. The conclusion is the testing procedures for eye examinations offer an examiner the ablity to establish an individual's specific optic requirements, to prescribe specific lenses, and to verify if the individual is wearing appropriate eyeglasses. However, unlike eye examintions, hearing tests do not offer the examiner the ability to establish an individual's specific amplification requirements, to prescribe a specific hearing aid for a particular hearing loss, or to verify if an individual is wearing the most appropriate hearing aid.

Proposing Medicare and other insurance programs pay for hearing aids when it is known there are no hearing tests available to establish an individual's specific amplification requirements or to verify if an individual is wearing the most appropriate hearing aid is unprincipled. The opportunity for abuse is enormous, and to propose only one professional group be eligible to perform those hearing tests and to dispense hearing aids for Medicare is equally unprincipled.

In addition to fostering professional solecism and chicanery, the flood of unregulated health and hospital insurance dollars into healthcare was creating social and economic problems. One social problem was the increasing number of individuals and employers who could no longer afford to purchase health and hospital insurance, and the difficulty those uninsured indviduals were having finding providers willing to offer them their services without payment. Insurance money had conjured the idea among too many providers they no longer had to provide their services without payment. An economic problem was the loss of many higher paying manufacturing jobs. The increasing cost of their employee's healthcare benefits was forcing many manufacturers to seek less expensive manufacturing opportunities outside of the United States.

If the United States is to retain its manufacturing economy, and if those manufactured products are to remain competitive in the present global economy, healthcare costs in the United States must be reduced to an internationally competitive 8–9% of the GNP.

A man who was one of my mentors possessed great vision. I recall his saying to me around 1970, "The problem with the public is they think in terms of the present rather than in terms of decades. Today, they are enjoying the unregulated services their insurance is purchasing for them, but they have given no thought to how the insurance they think is so wonderful today is going to destroy their healthcare delivery system in twenty years." He was right. Hopefully, this book will start people thinking about what could happen to the quality and the availability of their healthcare services in the next decade. Those quality and easily available services may no longer be available.

The Solution:
The solution for healthcare's escalating costs and for its service availability problems is the public's endorsement of the six changes to REGULATE the existing private healthcare delivery system. The six changes will reduce healthcare's costs by 25% to 30 % within two years and as much as 40% or more within five years. In addition, those reductions will provide our country an internationally competitive healthcare cost of only 8% to 9% of our GNP. Furthermore, the six changes will provide free outpatient and inpatient healthcare facilities to offer those individuals unable to pay for their services the opportunity to receive them.

3

Healthcare Legislation.

Prior to discussing the proposed six changes to regulate a private healthcare delivery system, the importance of healthcare legislation needs to be discussed. The public would be foolish not to consider the possibility of Congress passing legislation defining the future healthcare delivery system within this decade.

As will be repeatedly emphasized, the healthcare delivery system belongs to the public, and the power of their vote offers them the opportunity to insure legislation defining the future healthcare delivery system is favorable to them. But if the public is to use the power of their vote effectively, they must become informed political activists. Their elected represenatives in state legislatures and in Congress must be informed of the healthcare delivery system the public wants to have incorporated into legislation and of the public's willingness to use their vote to obtain that delivery system.

The delivery system the public must insist be incorporated into legislation is a regulated private healthcare delivery system. It offers the public their best opportunity to continue to receive comprehensive, quality, and easily available healthcare services as well as their best opportunity to attract the best from among our youth into healthcare. Fortunately, Congress failed to enact legislation establishing a National Health Service in the early 1990s. But without a challenge from an organized, informed, and politically active public, and without a solution for healthcare's cost and service availability problems, those lobbyists will succeed in obtaining favorable legislation for their clients within this decade. Furthermore, those lobbyists can expect support from the following:

1. Increasing public dependency on government.

2. The media.

3. Legislators.

4.   Special interests.

The Public's Dependency on Government:
Over the past forty years, many individuals in the United States have become dependent on, and conditioned to expect more from, government. Our country's income tax system illustrates why those individuals believe they can request more social programs from government without feeling threatened by the taxes required to fund those additional programs. In the United States, about 50% of the population pay about 94% of the income taxes, and the other 50% of the population pay only about 6% of those taxes. A tax increase to fund a National Health Service would not threaten the 50% of the population who pay only 6% of the income taxes. Also, the "free" healthcare services offered by such a delivery system would be attractive to them.

It is unfortunate those in government seeking the social transformation of our government, along with their accomplices in some of the media, can "use" those individuals who pay only 6% of the country's income taxes to advance their social agendas and to "use" the unfair graduated tax system in the United States to fund them. A legislator's awareness that 50% of the population will not object to increased taxes enables those legislators to have no concerns about proposing new and costly social programs to attract new voters and to increase the taxes necessary to fund them.

Unfortunately, the political rhetoric and the media have too many individuals mistakenly believing the existing graduated income tax code penalizes the "rich". It does not. Instead, it offers the "rich" many oportunities to shelter their wealth and incomes. More about this later.

As the public considers the advisability of a National Health Service as well as other social programs, they need to recall Professor Alexander Tyler's warning, circa 1778. "A democracy cannot exist as a permanent form of government. It can only exist until the voters discover that they can vote themselves largesse (generous gifts) from the public treasury."

The Media:
The cultural and social agendas of most of the TV network stations and most of the newspapers will prevent them from objectively reporting healthcare's issues. Those media outlets have compromised their journalistic intregity and objectivity, and they have lost their political neutrality. They have protrayed the United

States as imperialistic with racial and class oppression, and they have favored the Democratic political party. The following are a few examples.

Those media outlets protrayed the United States as the aggressor in Vietnam, and they have demeaned the soldiers who faught in that war. In contrast, the North Vietnamese, who had mudrered thousands to obtain their social and political agendas, were protrayed as victims. (September, 2003 issue of "The American Legion")

Those media outlets supported the resignation of one President for lying; however, the same media defended another President who had lied repeatedly.

Since 9/11, those same media outlets have been critical of the policies one President has taken to combat terrorism and to defend our national interests; however, the same media has been silent about another President's failure to initiate any meaningful action or policies to combat terrorism.

Those media outlets have opposed the appointment of qualified conservative judges to the federal judicial system; however, they have actively supported the appointment of judges who would support their more liberal social and political agendas.

Those media outlets are supporting those individuals who have been critical of the 87 billion dollar request to fund the war on terrorism, and they are demanding an accounting of where those dollars are to be spent. However, the same media has been silent about the 750 billion dollars the government spends to support the most expensive and the worst education system in the industrialized world, and they have never demanded an accounting of where those dollars are spent.

Those same media outlets have fostered the image of racial oppression and dependency in the United States. They have reported the political rhetoric that encourages many african-americans to beleive they are victims, and they have supported the welfare and other social programs that have kept too many people in political bondage. Hopefully, the african-american community will awaken and recognize that in 2003 everyone in the United States is born equally. It is what the person does with their life after birth that determines their quality of life. An individual does not help themselves by receiving fish. They help themselves by learning how to fish.

The same media's discussion of tax reform proposals has fostered class warfare in the United States. They have pitted the poor against the "rich", and the media has too many people mistakenly believing proposed tax reforms benefit the "rich". Mr. Forbes flat tax proposal is an example. Instead of benefiting the "rich", his flat tax would penalize the "rich". How? The existing tax codes offer the "rich" many opportunities to shelter their wealth and their incomes from taxation. For example, many individuals with incomes of $1,000,000 or more are known to pay less than 10% of their income in federal income taxes, or the individual with a million dollar income would pay less than $100,000 in income taxes. In contrast, an individual with an income of $100,000 could pay as much as 28% or more of their income in taxes, or their income tax would be $28,000 or more. It is obvious the existing tax codes favor the "rich". They pay much less in taxes relative to their incomes. However, if a 15% flat tax was the tax code with NO deductions, the "rich" would be penalized. The person with a $1,000,000 income would have to pay an income tax of $150,000. Their income tax would be increased by $50,000. In contrast, the individual making $100,000 would pay an income tax of $15,000. Their income tax would be reduced by $13,000.

Mr. Forbes's flat tax proposal, as well as other tax reform proposals, would have the "rich" paying much more of their wealth and incomes in taxes. However, the "rich" will do everything possible to have the public continue believing tax reform proposals benefit the "rich". It will discourage the public from supporting tax reform proposals that require them to pay more taxes. Also, with more objective alternative tax reporting, the media would be discussing the improved tax revenues Russia has obtained since they initiated a flat tax system similiar to Mr. Forbes.

The threat of the media to our country's future healthcare delivery system is the increasing number of people who do not think, question, or investigate. As Hitler's propagandist said, "If you repeat a lie enough times, most people will begin to believe it". Without an informed and questioning public, much of the media's reporting of healthcare issues can be expected to condition the public to support a National Health Service.

In fact, the conditioning process may have begun. In August of 2003, the Tampa Tribune printed an article from a national news source stating thousands of doctors favored a National Health Service. What the article did not say was the type of physician favoring the National Health Service. When the public considers the media's reporting of physician attitudes towards healthcare reforms, they need to remember there are three types of physicians. There are the several hundred thousand physicians who provide the public their medical and surgical services each day. A second group of physicians are the doctor's doctors. These are the physicians whose special skills are recognized by their colleagues and whose services they seek for themselves and for their families. The third type of physician is the administrative physician. These physicians have medical and osteopathic degrees, but they do not like to practice medicine or to treat patients. Instead, they have found administrative jobs in hospitals, HMOs, Medical Schools, and in federal and state government sponsored Public Health Services. If the reader had considered the Tampa Tribune's article in terms of the type of physician favoring the National Health Service, they would have discovered those thousands of doctors favoring a National Health Service were the administrative doctors. A National Health Service would offer them enormous job opportunities and power. The Department of Education is an example. Observe the number of administrative jobs available for educators in the Departments of Education in every state and in Washington, D.C., and observe the power those administrators possess. They establish the curriculum as well as other education policies for our country's public school system.

The Legislators:

Legislators are another reason why lobbyists seeking to replace the private delivery system may succeed. Too many legislators seek government as a career, and reelection becomes their primary mission. A union of the 50% of the public who pay little or no taxes with those individuals easily conditioned by the media to accept a National Health Service would form a formidable voting block driving legislators to endorse a National Health Service. Unfortunately, too many legislators sponsor and endorse legislation to win votes rather than to strengthen the defense and infrastructure of our country. A National Health Service would win many votes among the 50% or more of our population who pay few, or no, taxes.

Without public opposition, legislators will welcome the opportunity to pass legislation offering them control of the healthcare delivery system. Would their control be a problem for the public? Yes. The Department of Education is an example. Government has made the education system into a politically driven and expensive adminisrative bureaucracy, and the bureaucracy has provided our children the worst and the most expensive education among the industrialized nations. Furthermore, the money required to support the education bureaucracy is costing the taxpayors billions of dollars each year, and those dollars never reach the classroom. About 50% of the present 750 billion dollars required to fund the country's education system supports education's administrative bureaucracy. Legislators must never be allowed to do to the healthcare delivery system what they have done to the education system.

Special Interests Groups:
There are several special interests groups lobbying for favorable healthcare legislation, but only two are powerful enough to be considered a threat. One is the United States government, and the other is the managed healthcare industry (HMOs and multihospital companies).

Why should they be considered a threat? Both want to replace the private delivery system with one they can control. Control offers government enormous power. Think of the power government has obtained from the welfare voting blocks in every large city. A healthcare voting block would be much larger and more powerful. Furthermore, a government sponsored healthcare delivery system would increase public dependency on government, and this would be attractive to the socialists in our government. Control of healthcare would offer the managed healthcare industry easy profits.

Neither government nor the managed healthcare industry should be allowed to control healthcare. Neither can provide a delivery system better than the existing private delivery system, and neither possess the medical knowledge required to improve the services offered by the existing private delivery system.

Few with whom I have discussed the issue are aware of how a block of Congresspersons have been incrementally using legislation to achieve their goal of a National Health Service since the late 1950s. The idea of reproducing England's socialized healthcare delivery system in the United States was introduced in Congress during the late 1950s, but there was no public support. To introduce government into healthcare, Congress passed the Medicare and Medicaid legislation in the late 1960s. However, the absence of public support for goverment in healthcare continued. Most of the population were satistifed with their employer sponsored private health and hospital insurance and with the private healthcare delivery system. To achieve their goal of a National Health Service, Congress had to destroy both the private health insurance industry and the private healthcare delivery system. Both were successfully destroyed by legislation creating the HMO industry in the mid 1970s. (Addendum III)

The legislation provided HMOs the ablity to enroll only healthy individuals and to have relative immunity from lawsuits. Both provided HMOs the opportunity to offer the public less expensive premiums than those offered by competing indemnity insurance companies. Those less expensive premiums attracted many healthy individuals to the HMOs, and by the 1990s, the HMO industry, along with Medicare, had replaced the private insurance industry as the primary suppliers of, and payors for, healthcare's services. Furthermore, the private healthcare delivery system was being destroyed by the increasing HMO enrollments. Those increasing enrollments, along with Medicare's patients, became the majority of patients. To obtain patients, providers were forced to accept HMO and Medicare patients along with their mandated and unfriendly provider policies.

The successful use of the HMO industry to replace both the private insurance industry and the private healthcare delivery system required Congress to consider destroying the HMO industry if it was to achieve its goal of a National Health Service. The destruction of the HMO industry was planned with the proposed "Patient's Bill of Rights" legislation. The legislation would have had HMO enrollees suing their HMOs, and the cost of defending themselves from a flood of frivolous enrollee lawsuits would drive the HMO industry into bankruptcy. With an inactive private insurance industry and private healthcare delivery system, and with the HMO industry in bankruptcy, Congress would be "forced" to enact legislation creating a National Health Service. Hopefully, the "Patient's Bill of Rights" legislation as written now will never become law, and hopefully, neither government nor the managed healthcare industry will ever obtain control of healthcare.

The Problem of Disorganized Providers:
Many with whom I have spoken mistakenly believe organized medicine is a powerful lobby. They are wrong. Medical and Osteopathic Societies are no longer an organized and politically formidable professional lobbying group. Prior to the 1970s, those Societies were politically powerful. At the time, about 100% of practicing physicians were members of their local Medical Societies as well as the American Medical Association. Membership in those Societies was considered a requirement to practice medicine. Over the past thirty years, medicine has been fragmented into many different speciality organization, and the need for physicians to become members of those speciality organizations has replaced their need to become members of their local Societies and the American Medical Association. Also, each of those specialty groups has their own political aganda. Today, 40%, or less, of practicing physicians are members of either their local Societies

or the American Medical Association. Consequently, the political impact of those Societies has become insignificant.

I am in my late seventies, and I doubt if I will live into the next decade. However, the many reasons just discussed of why the lobbyists for government and the managed healthcare industry may obtain favorable healthcare legislation for their clients needs to be a concern for everyone. After my experiences as the Medical Director of an HMO, I can think of nothing worse for the public than legislation creating a government administered National Health Service whose healthcare services are offered by a profit driven managed healthcare company (HMO).

To be the beneficiary of future healthcare legislation, the public will have to recognize the many patient benefits offered them by the existing private healthcare delivery system, and they will have to recognize those benefits are worth preserving for themselves and for their families. Also, if the public chooses to preserve the private healthcare delivery system, they must offer their support to changing the existing private delivery system. It must be changed, and the public's endorsement of the proposed six changes to regulate a private healthcare delivery system will provide the necessary changes.

Is there a problem? Yes. The public does not appear to be aware of, or to feel threatened by, the loss of the private healthcare delivery system, and they have done nothing to support their physician's struggle to obtain favorable malpractice legislation.

As the public considers their need to participate in the legislative process to preserve a private healthcare delivery system, they need to observe the existing Department of Education. Think about the billions of healthcare dollars that will be required to support the administrative employees in both the federal and state Departments of Health who will be administering the National Health Service. Those billions of dollars will never be available to purchase healthcare services for the public. Also, if the HMO industry becomes the delivery system for the National Health Service, think of billions of healthcare dollars required to support the management and the operating expenses of the HMO industry. Again, those billions of dollars will never be available to purchase healthcare services for the public. Is this what the public wants?

The public must become aware of the importance of their role in the legislative process, and how legislation can impact negatively on them, and on their family's future. Learn about healthcare's antagonists—government and the managed healthcare industry. Both must be challenged if the legislative process is to be favorable to the public and to their families. Also, the public's elected representatives need to know of the public's willingnes to use their vote to insure a private healthcare delivery system is maintained.

If you remain undecided about your participation in the legislative process, you need to think of the possible alternative delivery systems legislation may impose on you in the next decade. The thought should frighten you.

4

Why Maintain a Private Healthcare Delivery System?

In addition to offering the public their best opportunity to continue to receive comprehensive, quality, and easily available healthcare services inexpensively, there are two additional reasons to maintain a regulated private healthcare delivery system. One is the inability of our country's economy to support the additional taxes required to fund a National Health Service. The other reason is to maintain a delivery system that offers physicians and other healthcare providers career incentives. The quality of the physicians providing a delivery system's services determines the quality of the servies offered by the delivery system.

The Economy:
Is it realistic to think our economy can support the additional taxes required to fund a politically and bureaucraticly driven National Health Service? At this time, the cost of government consumes a hugh 24% of our country's GNP, and during the past 40 years, the cost of government has been increasing faster than the rate of growth of the economy that supports it. The result has been increasing budget deficits, both federal and state. How much more can a government's growth continue to exceed the growth of the economy that supports it? Or, how much more tax money can government remove from the public to support additional government spending before the public's inability to purchase things causes a serious recession or depression? The public should keep in mind that history has shown socialism can not exist without a capitalistic economy to support its social programs. Is too much taxing destroying our capitalistic economy? Many economists say yes.

In 1946, I recall my college economics course taught me the public's ability to spend is the strength of a country's economy. When the public has money to spend, they buy "things", and their purchases generate sales taxes which benefit government. In addition, the public's purchases force manufacturers to produce more "things". Producing more "things" increases a manufacturer's profits, and those profits increase government's business tax revenues. Furthermore, producing more "things" requires manufacturers to employ more people. Those additional employed people receive an income, and they pay income taxes. Also, they purchase more "things" and generate more sales taxes. Both increase government's tax revenues.

In contrast, when taxes are increased, the public has less money to spend, and they stop purchasing "things". As fewer "things" are purchased, sales tax revenues decrease. Also, manufacturers are forced to reduce both their production and the number of their employees. The government loses business tax revenues as well as the loss of the unemployed's income taxes. Also, the unemployed have no extra money to spend to purchase "things", and this reduces the government's sales tax revenues. By increasing taxes, the government loses income taxes, sales taxes, and business taxes as well as causing many people to become unemployed.

Why is this fundamental economic principle so difficult for the public to understand. During the 1990s, our country had the largest state and federal government tax increases in its history. Those increasing taxes removed billions of dollars from the public's pockets, and those taxes reduced the public's purchasing power. The public's reduced purchasing power was a major cause of the economic decline and the increasing unemployment that began in 1998. Furthermore, the continuation of those taxes into the next decade and the continued reduction in the public's purchasing power will result in making the economic recovery from the present recession slower than it should be.

Again, I ask the question, "How much tax money can be removed from our economy before the economy collapses?" To ask the question another way, "Will removing more money from the public's pockets to provide the increased taxes required to support a National Health Service further reduce the public's purchasing power and initiate a significant economic slow down or depression in the United States? Most economists who are not politically dependent say yes. And, who gets hurt? The public! They would have increased taxes; they would have fewer jobs available; and they would be dissatisfied with the services offered by a National Health Service.

Is it possible the adoption of a National Health Service and the increased taxes required to support it is the plan of the socialists in our government? It would create more unemployment and more public dependency on government. Both are attractive to socialists.

The public should remind themselves the taxing power of our government was intended to enable the government to fund the country's defense and to fund the building and maintenance of its infrastructure. Why has the government's spending priorities and the most expensive budget items become the many government sponsored social programs? Of course, to increase the public's dependency on government and to obtain votes. The public should not allow a National Health Service to become another of those expensive social programs.

Provider Career Incentives:
The other reason for maintaining a regulated private healthcare delivery system is to provide the career incentives necessary to attract the best from among our youth into healthcare. Over the past thirty years, neither government's (Medicare) nor the managed healthcare industry's (HMOs) policies have been provider friendly. They have offered providers no career incentives, and they have forced providers to comply with unnecessary regulations and documentation requirements. Too many physicians no longer find practicing medicine enjoyable, and many are anxious for their children to complete their education so they can retire. Also, they no longer recommend medicine as a career, and the number of applicants for admission into Medical Schools is declining. Why spend ten to fifteen years at great expense studying to become a physician whose future is an employee of a National Health Service or of a managed healthcare company (HMO)?

Is the public aware of the importance of the physician to the quality and availability of their future healthcare services? The public is reminded of the difference between being offered their services and being provided their services. Any delivery system can offer the public their medical and surgical services; however, only a physician can provide those services. Furthermore, the quality of those services will depend on the quality of the physicians providing them, and the availablity of those services will depend on the number of physcians available to provide them. Without career incentives, the best from among our youth will no longer be attracted to healthcare, and the numbers of those entering healthcare will continue to decline.

When thinking about healthcare issues, the public is encouraged to think about them in terms of decades. For example, training a physician requires more than ten years. If the public discovers in the next decade they are dissatisfied with the quality and availability of their physicians, it will take another decade to produce more physicians. Therefore, it becomes incumbent on the public to insure the future healthcare delivery system offers physicians career incentives. Without them, the best from among our youth will not be attracted into healthcare.

A regulated private healthcare delivery system offers the public their best opportunity to provide physicians career incentives. They are:

a. the opportunity to be independent practitioners in a fee-for-service private delivery system rather than an employee of a National Health Service or of a managed healthcare company (HMO).

b. the opportunity to receive reimbursements for their services established by a standard (Provider Reimbursement Formula) rather than reimbursements arbitarily established by a third party.

c. the opportunity to have ALL healthcare dollars spent purchasing healthcare services rather than spent supporting the administrative bureaucracy of another government social program or the management and operational costs of a managed healthcare company.

d. the opportunity to treat patients who have had the freedom to select the providers of their choice.

e. the opportunity to determine their patient's needs, independent of a third party's approval.

f. the opportunity to offer their patients more comprehensive, better quality, and more easily available services, at a lower cost than those offered by either an HMO or a National Health Service.

The quality and the availability of the services offered by any delivery system depend on its physicians. Attracting the best from among our youth to become those physicians will depend on the career incentives offered to them. Forcing physicians to become employees of either a National Health Service or of a managed healthcare company will not be attractive career incentives.

5

Legislation and the Public's Complacency.

Some form of legislation defining the future healthcare delivery system appears to be inevitable within the next decade. To think otherwise would be foolish. The government's investment in Medicare as well as the damaging impact the increasing cost of healthcare is having on our economy will encourage such legislation. Will the legislation provide the public a delivery system whose services possess the quality, the comprehensiveness, and the availability of the services offered by the existing private healthcare delivery system?

If I were asked to identify a serious healthcare problem, I would have to identify the public's complacency about healthcare legislation. Healthcare legislation will influence how our youth views healthcare as a career opportunity. Is the public's silence about supporting their physician's efforts to enact malpractice reform legislation a reflection of their indifference to the importance of physicians in their future healthcare delivery system? Has the public mistakenly assumed physicians who have come from the best of our youth will be there in the next decade? Has a misinformed public assumed the "government" will be there to offer them their healthcare services in the next decade? True, the government may be offering their healthcare services, but who will be providing those services?

Instead of the public focusing their healthcare concerns on who will be paying for their healthcare services, they need to focus on who will be providing those services. Insurance will remain the payment system for healthcare's services regardless of the delivery system offering them. However, the quality of, and the number of, the physicians providing those services may not be the same in the next decade, or for decades to come.

Once again! Any delivery system can offer the public their healthcare services, but only physicians along with other healthcare providers can provide those services. Once again, the quality of those services will depend on the quality of the providers who provide them, and the availability of those services will depend on the number of providers available to provide them.

As your thoughts wonder into the next decade and how healthcare legislation could impact on your life, and your family's life, ask yourself these questions:

1. Am I going to be satisfied when my healthcare services become increasingly more difficult to obtain?

2. Am I going to be satisfied when a third party tells me when, where, and from whom I will receive my services?

3. Am I going to be satisfied when the quality and comprehensiveness of my services become inferior to the quality of the services I'm now receiving?

4. Am I going to be satisfied when my services are no longer provided by providers who have come from among the best of our youth?

5. Am I going to be satisfied when a politically driven and bureaucratically administered government sponsored National Health Service offers me my services from the lowest-bid managed healthcare company?

6. Or, are the many benefits I have received from the private healthcare delivery system worth preserving?

Can the public acknowledge the importance of the physician in healthcare? Will the public participate in obtaining legislation offering the career opportunities necessary for our youth to consider becoming future physicians? Or, will the legislation favor the politician by endorsing a National Health Service and favor the investors in managed healthcare companies by having them become the delivery system for the National Health Service?

As I see it, it is the public vs. the government and investors. Who is going to be the winner?

6

The Proposed Six Changes To Regulate a Private Delivery System.

Opposition to the proposed six changes to regulate a private healthcare delivery system can be expected from some patients and from some providers as well as from most attorneys. However, the six changes are not proposed to benefit either individual patients, providers, or attorneys. Instead, they are proposed to benefit the public by insuring the many patient benefits offered by a regulated private healthcare delivery system are maintained.

Can the necessary reductions in the cost of healthcare's services be achieved in a private healthcare delivery system? And, can the existing service availability problems for those unable to pay for their services be corrected in a private healthcare delivery system?

The answer to both questions is yes. The proposed six changes address the four major causes for healthcare's increasing costs. Two of the four causes are the costs associated with patients receiving medically unnecesary services and the costs of the increase physician and other provider fees. The third cause is the cost associated with frivlous malpractice litigation, and the fourth cause is the cost associated with the administrative expenses required to comply with the many unnecessary regulations and documentation requirements of Medicare and the HMO industry.

All four of those costs are addressed by the proposed six changes to regulate a private healthcare delivery system. They introduce price controls to control the cost of healthcare's services; they introduce more effective monitoring to control the medical necessity of the services patients receive; they introduce litigation reforms to control litigation costs; and, by preserving the private healthcare delivery system, many of the expensive and unnecessary HMO and Medicare regulations and documentation requirements are eliminated.

In addition, the six changes address the service availability problem for those unable to purchase their medical and surgical services. Free heathcare facilities like those that existed prior to the 1970s will be opened.

Equally important, the six changes return the responsibility for controlling the professional behavior of physicians to local Medical and Osteopathic Societies; they return the responsibility for monitoring the medical necessity of the services patients receive to those Societies; and they return the responsibility for judging the merit of malpractice lawsuits to those Societies.

The six changes to regulate a private healthcare delivery system are:

1. Changing how a provider's reimbursement is calculated.

2. Copayments.

3. Monitoring for the medical necessity of the services patients are receiving.

4. Regulating allowable hospital fixed costs and monitoring hospital variable costs

5. Reforming the litigation process.

6. Establishing free outpatient and inpatient healthcare facilities.

7

Changing How a Provider's Reimbursement is Calculated.

The first of the six changes to regulate the private healthcare delivery system is changing how the reimbursements for all of healthcare's providers are calculated.

After three decades of adjusting to arbitrarily established provider reimbursements by the HMO industry and Medicare, few physicians will question the importance of a maintaining a fee-for-service private healthcare delivery system in which their reimbursements are calculated by a standard. This is possible if the six changes to regulate a private healthcare delivery system are endorsed.

Perhaps the most difficult of the six changes for some physicians to accept is the change in how their reimbursements are calculated. Their reimbursements may be less than their present reimbursements. However, all physicians will be receiving generous reimbursements for their services and for their office expenses. In addition, those reimbursement will insure the preservation of the private healthcare delivery system. A private delivery system is the best delivery system for the professional future of existing physicians, and for the future of those physicians to follow them.

The following are the four changes in how provider reimbursements are to be calculated.

1. The first change is to stop "relative value" payments. The relative value payment system became popular during the 1970s to justify the increasing number of medically unnecessary services being offered to patients. The more valuable a service was considered to be in the diagnosis and treatment of a disorder or disease the larger its insurance reimbursement.

No service has a "relative value". A service is either necessary or it is not necessary, and if physicians want a private delivery system, they need to possess the leadership required to identify unnecessary services and to eliminate their insurance reimbursements.

2. The second change is to stop awarding insurance payments for medically unnecessary services.

After my retirement, I became the Medical Director of an HMO for a short period of time. During that time, I was able to identify at least 30% of the services requested by, or offered to, our enrollees to be medically unnecessary. Those unnecessary services created enormous healthcare costs.

The monitoring for medical necessity recommendations contained in the third change to regulate a private healthcare delivery system will offer physicians the opportunity to identify medically unnecessary services and to eliminate the need for insurance to offer reimbursements for them.

Although a service has been identified as medically unnecessary, patients may continue to receive the service; however, their insurance will no longer pay for the service.

3. The third change in how provider reimbursements are awarded is to stop the larger reimbursements for procedure services. It takes the same amount of training, knowledge, and skill to become a physician who offers no procedure services (Internists, Family Physicians, and Pediatricians) as it does to become a physician who offers procedure services (Surgeons). Accordingly, their reimbursements should be the same.

The proposed change awards all necessary medical and surgical services the same reimbursements calculated by the Provider Reimbursement Formula.

The present higher incomes offered by some specialities have attracted physicians to those specialities. When young physicians consider speciality training opportunities, their consideration should focus on their interest in the speciality rather than on the income offered by the speciality.

4. The Provider Reimbursment Formula is the fourth change in how the insurance reimbursements for all providers are to be calculated. The Formula has three components. They are:

A. The cost of the provider.

All of healthcare's providers are assigned an hourly payment rate for their services, and it will be adjusted annually based on inflation.

A physician's hourly rate is $200/hour. (The physician's rate was suggested in 1988 when the Provider Reimburement Formula was introduced, and it will require revision based on an appropriate inflation formula.)

B. The time required to complete the service.

The time required to complete all services is established, and the Formula refers to it as the "service time".

To determine if a provider's "service time" reimbursement requests are appropriate, all offices will be required to maintain a daily log of the patients served and their diagnosis.

C. The office overhead allowance.

The Formula includes an insurance reimbursement for a provider's office overhead expenses in addition to their "service time" reimbursement. The office overhead expenses will vary in different parts of the country and with different specialities.

The office overhead allowance is calculated by establishing the time an office is available to offer patients services and by the amount of money the Formula allows a provider for their annual office expenses.

Office availability is established by accepting every office to be available to patients 40hr./week and for 44 weeks each year. This amounts to 1750 hours of office availability annually. (8 weeks a year are allowed for a provider's vacation and meeting/education attendence.)

The office overhead allowance is based on the "service time" required to complete the service, and the methodology to establish the allowable office expenses exists.

Examples of the Provider Reimbursement Formula.

The following five examples illustrate how easily the Formula can be applied to calculate the insurance reimbursements for all services. In each of the examples, the dollars are 1988 dollars. Although small increases will be necessary, an appropriate inflation formula needs to be applied to raise the dollars to 2003 dollars.

A.   All providers are physicians who receive $200/hour for their service time. If a provider offers services for at least 1750 hours (40hr./week for 44 weeks), the provider's insurance reimbursements for the "service time" would be $350,000. In addition to their "service time" reimbursement, the provider receives an office overhead allowance based on the "service time".

B.   The office overhead allowance (OOA) in each of the examples was calculated to be $54/hour for each hour of "service time", and it was calculated as follows:

The office availability for each provider is 40hr./week for 44 weeks each year, or 1750 hours of office availability annually. The amount of money each of the providers in the five examples is allowed for their annual office expenses is $95,000. A provider can spend more money than the Formula allows for their offices, but their insurance reimbursement will be calculated on the Fomula's allowance.

By dividing 1750 hours of office availability time into the $95,000 allowed for the annual office expenses, a $54/hour office overhead payment for each hour of "service time" is obtained for each of the following five examples.

The office overhead allowance in not restricted to services offered in an office. It is offered for services provided patients outside of the office, such as operations. An office must be maintained while a provider is offering services such as surgery outside of their office.

Example One.

Example one is a surgical procedure whose present charge is $6,000. Applying the Provider Reimbursement Formula (PRF), the insurance reimbursement for this operation is:

1.   The cost of the provider:

The provider is a physician who receives $200/hour of service time.

2.   The time required to complete the service:

a.   Complete the preoperative hospital records - 30 min.

b.   Time to complete the operation - - - - - - - - 3 1/2 hr.

c.   Time to complete the post operative records - 15 min.

d.   Daily post operative visits - - - - - - - - - - - - 1 1/2 hrs.

The patient's LOS (length of stay) for this operation is six days with two daily visits: one for 10 min. and another for 5 min, for a total of 11/2 hrs. for the six days.

e.   Time to complete discharge records - - - - - - - 15 min.

The Formula allows a "service time" of 6 hrs. to complete this operation, and the surgeon's "service time" reimbursement is $1,200. (6 hrs X $200/hr.)

3.   The Office Overhead Allowance.(OOA)

The office overhead allowance (OOA) for this surgeon is $54/hr. for each hour of "service time". The OOA is $340 (6 hrs. X $54) for this operation.

The Formula's reimbursement for this operation is $1, 524. ($1,200 for the "service time" + $324 for the OOA). The Formula saves $4,460 each time this operartion is performed. (Present charge of $6,000, and the PRF's reimbursement is $1,524.)

Example Two.

The second example is an office procedure whose present charge is $850. Applying the PRF, the provider's reimbursement is calculated as follows:

1.   The cost of the provider:

a.   The provider is a physician who receives $200/hr. of service time.

b.   In this example, a technician's assistance is required. The techician is a salaried employee and the Formula allows $30/hr. for salary and benefits.

2.   The time required to complete the service:

a.   To review the patient's chart and
complete the necessary records - - - - - 20 min.

b.   To perform the procedure - - - - - - - - - 20 min.

   c.   To discuss the results with the patient
       and complete necessary records - - - - - 20 min.

The Formula allows one hour of "service time" for this service, and the "service time" insurance reimbursement is $230. (The physician's reimbursement is $200, and the technician's reimbursement is $30.)

3.   The Office Overhead Allowance (OOA);

   This physician's OOA is $54 for each hour of "service time". The Formula's OOA for this procedure is $54. (1 hr. of "service time" X $54)

   Special Overhead Allownaces:

   Special office overhead allowances are offered for equipment, medications, and instruments used in completing a service. Their reimbursement is calculated on their purchase and maintenance costs and on their depreciation. For this procedure the special equipment allowance is $25 each time the procedure is performed.

The total Office Overhead Allowance for this procedure is $79. ($54 for one hour of "service time" and $25 for the equipment allowance.)

The total insurance reimbursement for this office procedure is $309. (Provider's "service time" is $230, and the OOA is $79.)

Each time this procedure is performed the Formula saves $541. (Present charge is $850, and the formula's reimbursement is $309)

Example Three.

This procedure is performed in both a physician's office and in outpatient surgical centers. The present charge is about $1,000. Applying the Formula to calculate the insurance reimbursement for this procedure:

1.   The cost of the provider.

   The provider is a physician who receives $200 for each hour of "service time".

2. The time to complete the service:

    a. To complete the patient's records and
        prepare the patient for the procedure - - - - 15 min.

    b. To complete the procedure - - - - - - - - - - - 15 min.

    c. To give the patient their postoperative
        instructions and complete their records - - - 15 min.

    The Formula allows a 45 minute "service time" for this procedure, and the Formula's "service time" reimbursement is $150. (3/4s of an hour X $200.)

3. The office overhead allowance.

    The Formula allows an OOA of $54 for each hour of "service time". The OOA for this procedure is $42. (3/4s of an hour X $54.)

The total reimbursement for this procedure is $192. (The "service time" reimbursement is $150, and the OOA is $42.)

The Formula saves $808 each time this procedure is performed.

Example Four.

The fourth example of the Provider Reimbursement Formula is its application to calculate the insurance reimbursements for office visits.

The Formula recognizes five types of office visits.

1. 0 to 5 minutes

2. 5 to 10 minutes.

3. 10 min. to 15 min.

4. 15 min. to 20 min.

5. 20 min. or more

Applying the Formula to calculate the reimbursement for a five minute office visit:

1. The cost of the provider.

    The provider is a physician who receives $200/hour for their "service time".

2. The time required to complete the service:

    There are twelve 5 minutes in each hour. Divide 12 into $200, and each 5 minute office visit receives a $17 "service time" reimbursement.

3. The office overhead allowance.

    The office overhead allowance is $54 for each hour of "service time". The office overhead allowance for a 5 minute office visit is $5. (Divide12 into $54/hour of "service time".)

The Formula's reimbursement for a five minute office visit is $22 ($17 is for the "service time" + $5 is for the Office Overhead Allowance.

The following are the Formula's reimbursements for the other four types of office visits including both the "service time" and the Office Overhead Allowances.
5–10 min. $42. ($33 for "service time" + $9 for the OOA)
10–15 min. $64. ($50 for "service time" + $14 for the OOA)
15–20 min. $85. ($67 for "service time" + $18 for the OOA)
20min. or more $127 ($100 for "service time" + $27 for the OOA)

The duration of an office visit will vary according to the disease or disorder being treated. In most instances, the time a physician spends with a patient is within 10 minutes.
However, there are many office visits lasting less than five minutes. These visits are not infreqent, and they are for the physician to quickly check to be sure everything is progressing satisfactorily.

An example of the Formula's savings is a recent office charge of $78. The physician was with the patient only seven minutes. The Formula would have paid the physician only $42 (a 5–10 minute office visit) instead of the $78, and the Formula would have saved $36.

Recording the number of office visits and the time for each visit is easily accomplished with existing insurance company computers. An example of a possible problem is a physician's request for insurance reimbursements for six hours of "service time", but only eight patients were treated. The problem could be either overcharging, taking too much time with each patient, or the complexity of the problem. Another example of a possible insurance abuse is a patient having four consecutive office visits lasting within ten minutes for disease Y when the usual standard is only one initial ten minute office visit and one quick 5 minute follow-up office visit.

Example Five.

The fifth example of the Provider Reimbursement Formula is the reimbursements for hospital consultations. Both the number of unnecessary hospital consultations as well as the frequency of physician visits following the initial consultation create unnecessary costs. Those consultations need to be monitored for their medical necessity.

The Formula will reimburse only two types of hospital visits.

a. For an initial consultation, the formula offers a $127.00 reimbursement (a 20 minute or more visit).

b. For the visits following the initial consultation, the Formula offers a $42 reimbursement for the first visit and $22 for each visit thereafter.

No examples of how the Provider Reimbursement Formula calculates the reimbursements for Xray and other diagnostic studies is presented, but the Formula does provide significant savings for those studies. For example, the reimbursement for Xrays would be calculated as follows.

1. The cost of the providers:

a. A physician who receives $200/hour of "service time".

b. A technician who receives $X/hour of "service time".

2. The time required to complete the service.

The time reqired to complete the service for the physician is the time required to read the Xrays, to dictate a report, and to review and sign the report of the Xray. The time for the technician is the time require for the technician to take the particular Xray. Some Xrays will require the physicians's participation as well.

3. The Office Overhead Allowance is based on the cost of the equipment require to take the particular Xray, and the cost of the personnel required to maintain the office and to maintain the equipment.

The examples illustrate how the proposed Provider Reimbursement Formula offers all physicians and other providers equal, as well as generous, compensation for their services. However, the Formula's reimbursements are not arbitrarily established. They are established by a standard that is applied to all services.

The Formula introduces price controls, and most physicians will accept those price controls as long as they offer them and other providers career incentives. This subject is discussed in Addendum I.

8

Patient Copayments.

The second change to regulate the private healthcare delivery system is the use of copayments for office visits and hospital consultations.

Yes, copayments are necessary. When "something" is considerd to be "free", individuals disregard both the need for the "something" as well as its cost. Since health and hospital insurance, rather than the patient's pocketbook, will remain the primary source of payment for healthcare's services, copayments have become necessary to encourage patients to think about the need for, as well as the cost of, their services.

There are many individuals in the United States who have acquired the "entitlement" mentality. They believe they are entitled to receive all of their services without their need to pay for them, and those individuals can be expected to challenge copayments. However, patients are reminded. Their copayments will contribute to preserving the private healthcare delivery system with its many patient benefits.

Copayments are not new. The managed healthcare industry has had copayments since its inception, and most pharmacy insurance plans require copayments. Furthermore, copayments are being discussed in Congress for Medicare patients.

Copayments will become part of any future healthcare delivery system, but the public will benefit most if the copayments are part of a regulated private healthcare delivery system rather than part of either a National Health Service or an HMO.

The suggested copayments for office visits are: (1988 dollars)

    a.   0 to 5 minutes - - - - - - - - - - - - $5

    b.   5–15 min. office visit - - - - - - $10

c.   15–20 min. office visit- - - - - - $20

d.   20 min. or more office visit - - $30

In addition to the copayments for office visits, copayments are necessary for both initial hospital consultations and for the physician visits following the initial consultation. Both generate unnecessary costs, and copayments will motivate patients to question the medical necessity of them.

The suggested copayment for an initial hospital consultation is $30, and the suggested copayment for all of the visits following the initial consultation is $5.

There will be copayments for some diagnostic studies. Also, copayment adjustments will be necessary for both Medicaid and some Medicare patients but the services these patients receive will be closely monitored for their medical necessity.

Patients will pay their copayment directly to their provider, and the provider will deduct the patient's copayment from their request for their insurance reimbursements. For example, the Formula allows $127 for an initial hospital consultation. The patient's copayment is $30. The provider will collect the $30 copayment from the patient, and he, or she, will request a $97 insurance reimbursement.

9

Monitoring for Medical Necessity

The third change to regulate the private healthcare delivery system is monitoring the services patients receive for their medical necessity.

The "free" services provided by unregulated health and hospital insurance programs have encouraged patients to request, and providers to offer, medically unnecessary services. To eliminate the significant costs associated with those unnecessary services, monitoring the services patients receive for their medical necessity has become a requirement. Furthermore, the Provider Reimbursement Formula introduces price controls, and those controls could encourage some providers to offer medically unnecessary services to compensate for the price controls. If patients want insurance to pay for their services, and if providers want the security of insurance reimbursements for their services, both will have to acknowledge the need for insurance companies to monitor the medical necessity of the services they purchase.

What is a medically necessary service?

a. The service has to have a documented medical value, and

b. The service has to be necessary to either diagnosis or treat the disorder or disease.

As the Medical Director of an HMO, I was able to identify at least 30% of the services our HMO enrollees were receiving to be medically unnecessary. Based on those HMO experiences, individuals making medical necessity decisions can expect to encounter four problems. The first problem will be the qualification of the individual making the decisions. No individual possess the knowledge necessary to make medical necessity decisions about all of the different services patients require to diagnosis or to treat the many different diseases and disorders. To properly assess the medical necessity of patient services, more than one individual is required to make medical necessity decisions. The second problem is making medical necessity decisions before the patient receives the service. Those decisions should never be made before the patient receives the service. Too frequently, patients have been denied a necessary service prior to their receiving it, and their treatment has been compromised. All medical necessity decisons must be made after the patient has received the service. The third problem is the need to identify a service as medically unnecessary even though it has a known medical value. An example is the use of an antibiotic to treat a virus infection. Antibiotics have a known medical value. They destroy bacteria. However, antibiotics do not destroy virus. Therefore, when an antibiotic is used to treat a common cold (viral infection), it is medically unnecessary. But, when an antibiotic is used to treat a bacterial complication of a viral infection, the antibiotic is medically necessary. The fourth problem is the need to identify a service as possessing no medical value. At the present time, patients are receiving, and insurance is paying for, services that have no known medical value. Eliminating the insurance reimbursements for these services will initiate legal challenges, and because of those legal issues, those services will not be identified at this time. Nevertheless, they need to be identified, and their insurance reimbursements stopped.

Monitoring for medical necessity is not new; however, it has not been effective for several reasons:

1. Monitoring by unqualified individuals.

2. The absence of penalities for those individuals offering and requesting unnecesary services.

3. Litigation issues.

    a. A provider's fear of being sued for not having offered a service, and

    b. A providers fear of being sued by those whose services they are monitoring.

Monitoring by Unqualified Individuals:
To evaluate the medical necessity of the services Medicare and Medicaid patients were receiving, the government awarded contracts to individuals to establish Peer Review Organizations, referred to as the PROs. The PROs employed physicians and other providers to monitor the services Medicare and Medicaid patients were receiving. Based on my experiences with the PROs, many of those individuals

employed by the PROs were not qualified to monitor the services they were directed to monitor. For example, a surgeon is not capable of making medical necessity judgements about all the many different surgical services. One experience among several of mine was a PRO representative denying ten days of hospitalization for a patient of mine who had had extensive surgery for cancer with reconstruction of the mouth and throat. The patient had difficulty learning to swallow following the surgery, and their hospitalization was prolonged. When I attended the PRO's appeals hearing, I learned the individual who had monitored my patient's services and who had denied the ten days of hospitalization had never performed a surgical procedure like the one I had performed. Furthermore, when asked, the individual was unable to descirbe the physiology of swallowing. Regardless of his inadequate knowledge of the operation, of the physiology of swallowing, and of the patient's recovery problems, the hospital was denied ten days of Medicare reimbursements for my patient. This is an example of how, among several of my experiences, the PRO's mission was to demonstrate to the government they could save Medicare money rather than to objectively evaluate the medical necessity of the services Medicare's patients were receiving.

The proposed changes in medical necessity monitoring will replace the PROs with local Medical and Osteopathic Society Monitoring Teams. Local Socieites are preferred to the PROs for several reasons. Perhaps the most important is their ability to provide the most qualified providers to monitor the services of another provider. Also, all services patients receive, not only Medicare's and Medicaid's, will be monitored, and monitoring by local Societies will be less expensive than the PROs,

Prior to the 1970s, local Medical and Osteopathic Societies effectively monitored the professional activities of community physicians. For example, in 1961, I had to appear before a local Society's ethics review board to defend my insertion of tubes into children's ears. There was a complaint from other physicians who were not inserting the tubes. I successfully defended the surgical procedure; however, at that time, I could have been censured and possibly lost my license to practice medicine. But today, the existing litigation system would offer me the opportunity to stop the investigation by initiating a lawsuit against the Society,

Unfortunately, since litigation became such a dominant force in our culture, physicians whose services were being investigated have been able to stop the investigation by initiating a lawsuit against the Society and sometimes against the provider who is monitoring their services. The Society is forced to stop the investigation because the Society, as well as the individual performing the monitoring, would have to employ an attorney to defend themselves. The problem is not the cost of the attorneys. The problem is neither the Society nor the monitoring physician would be able to recover any of their attorney's fees or other defense costs after they successfully defend themselves against the lawsuit.

When I have told individuals about the inability of the medical profession to police the professional activities of community physicians, their response is always, "The Society would win the lawsuit. What is the problem?" Of course the Society would win the lawsuit, but the public has no understanding of the cost of defense. Since the public can initiate a lawsuit without any cost to themselves, they forget those being sued have the expense of emoloying an attorney to defend themselves. For example, if a local Society were to initiated investigations of ten physicians, and if five of those physicians were to initiate lawsuits against the Society, the cost of engaging the attorneys necessary to defend the Society would be enormous. Although the Society would win those lawsuits, the Society would not be able to recover any of their legal defense expenses after successfully defending themselves. However, there is a solution for a Society's inability to recover its defense expenses. The solution is the "loser pays all" policy. This policy is discussed in the fifth change to regulate a private healthcare delivery system.

The proposed change in medical necessity monitoring would establish a Medical Necessity Monitoring Committee in every local Medical and Osteopathic Society. Those Committees would replace the PROs. When the Society receives a medical necessity monitor request from an insurance company, or from any other source, the Society's Monitoring Committee would appoint at least two physicians to a monitoring Team. Those two physicians would offer the same service as those to be monitored. The Team members would evaluate the medical necessity of the service in question, and they would send their report to the Society's Monitoring Committee. If the Team had found the service to be medically unnecessary, the Society's Monitoring Committee would offer an invitation to the provider and to the patient to appear before the Comittee and appeal the medical necessity decision before the Committee decided upon any action.

Team members would be compensated by the insurance company requesting the monitor, and the compensation would be calculated by the Provider Reimbursement Formula.

All community providers would be obligated to accept assignments to their local Society's Monitoring Teams regardless of whether or not they were members of those Societies. If a provider fails to accept an assignment, there will be penalities, such as losing their ability to collect insurance reimbursements for their services from the insurance company requesting the monitor for a specified period of time.

All monitors would be done after the patient has recevied the service. A physician's recommended treatment program will not be compromised by making medical necessity judgements prior to the patient receiving the service.

In addition to the ability of local Medical and Osteopathic Society Monitoring Teams to improve the quality and the effectiveness of medical necessity monitoring, the proposed Monitoring Teams would be less expensive. An example is a newspaper advertisement (Philadelphia Inquirer, Sept., 2000). The Independence Blue Cross stated they had 30 medical doctors and 250 registered nurses on staff making medical necessity decisions about the services their members were receiving. The Blue Cross monitoring policy is an excellent policy. It provides public safety and reduces the cost of unnecessary services, but it is more expensive than a Society's monitoring Team.

If the decision of a local Society's Team is challenged by the provider being investigated, the provider can request another Society's Team monitor the medical necessity of their service. However, the provider would have to pay the cost of the monitor.

The Absence of Penalties:
The second reason why medical necessity monitoring has been unsuccessful is the absence of penalties for those patients who go from provider to provider requesting unnecessary services and for those providers who offer those unnecessary services.

The penalities must be severe. The suggested penalties for providers would be the need to repay the insurance reimbursements for the unnecessary service. In addition, depending on the severity and frequency of the insurance abuses, additional penalties could range from fines to a provider's inability to receive insurance reimbursements from a specific company for a specified period of time. The charge of fraud is possible.

The penalities for patients who go from provider to provider requesting unnecessary services could range from increasing their copayments to their inablity to use their insurance to pay for a specified service for a period of time.

Litigation and monitoring:
The third reason why past medical necessity monitoring has been unsuccessful is our country's out-of-control litigation system. Physicians are forced to offer their patients unnecessary services to protect themselves from frivolous malpractice lawsuits. Physicians know attorneys focus more on what the attorney is able to convince a jury the physician should have done rather than what the physician did. Accordingly, physicians order many unnecessary services to protect themselves in case their patient initiates a malpractice lawsuit. The only way to eliminate the need for physicians to order unnecessary services to protect themselves from frivolous lawsuits is to endorse the "loser pays all" policy. (The fifth change to regulate a private healthcare delivery system.)

An additional litigation problem for medical necessity monitoring is the problem encountered by those monitoring the services of others. Not infrequently, the physician investigating the services of another is sued by the provider they are investigating. The combination of the cost of employing an attorney to defend themselves and the inability to recover any of their attorney's fees or other defense costs when they successfully defend themselves is the reason physicians frequently refuse to monitor the services of other physicians. An example is my experience as the Medical Director of an HMO. I had questioned a physician's surgical procedure and his fee. The response to my inquiry was a letter from the physician stating if I continued with these questions, his professional standing in the community could be threatened as well as his patient/physician relationship. He would be forced to seek legal counsel if my questions continued. A potential lawsuit was directed at me. Since the organization I was representing did not wish to pay for my defense, my inquiry into the physician's service and fee was dropped. I had no question about my ability to defend myself successfully, but there would be no way for me to recover my attorney's expenses and other defense costs after the lawsuit.

Few, if any, physicians will be willing to monitor the services of other physicians without protection from lawsuits. The problem is not the lawsuit. The problem is the inability of those being sued to recover any of their attorney's fees or other defense costs after they have successfully defended themselves.

The public's endorsement of the litigation changes proposed in the fifth change to regulate a private healthcare delivery system is essential if medical necessity monitoring is to be successful.

Achieving successful medical necessity monitoring will not be easily accomplished. Over the past thirty years, patients have been receiving services that have had questionable medical values, and both physicians and patients can be expected to challenge an insurance company's request to have those services monitored for their medical necessity. Accordingly, medical necessity monitoring will require both strong leadership within Medical and Oeteopathic Societies and protection from frivolous lawsuits. The former will require physician support, and the latter will require the public's support. The public's vote is the tool necessary to build a concensus among legislators that litigation reforms favoring the public are necessary.

10

Regulating Hospital Costs.

The fourth change to regulate the private healthcare delivery system is the regulation of a hospital's allowable fixed costs and the monitoring of its variable costs.

Prior to the 1950s, hospitals were charitable community institutions providing services to all in need of those services regardless of their ability to pay. Those patients who could afford to pay for their services paid for them from their pocketbooks. Those who could not afford to purchase their services were able to obtain them in their local hospital's free inpatient wards. However, as more and more individuals obtained hospital insurance, the need for free hospital facitilities decreased, and by the 1970s, the free hospital inpatient wards had closed. Hospital insurance had replaced the patient's pocketbook as the primary source of payment for hospital services.

Regretably, those insurance programs failed to challenge either unnecessary hospital admissions or the increasing charges for, and the medical necessity of, hospital services. Patients were hospitalized unnecessarily, the charges for many hospital services increased, and both physicians and patients became indifferent to the medical necessity of hospital services. These insurance abuses were generating billions of insurance dollars, and as those dollars flowed into the hospital system, hospitals became profitable. Those profits attracted businesspersons with their investors, and during the 1970s, for-profit and investor owned multihospital management companies began to appear. Over the past several decades, those companies have transformed the charitable community hospital system into an insurance driven, for-profit, multihospital business system.

Both a hospital's fixed and its variable costs can be reduced significantly. If I were asked, I would estimate those costs could be reduced by at least a 30–35% within five years.

Fixed costs are costs always present regardless of how many patients are in a hospital, and those costs can be reduced by regulating the amount of money a hospital is allowed to apply to each patient's daily charges for its fixed costs. The following are examples of a hospital's fixed costs that can be reduced or eliminated.

1. Construction costs.

    Hospitals construction goals need to focus on a patient's service requirements rather than on asthetics. When one enters a hospital they should not think of themselves as entering a luxury hotel.

    During the 1950s and 1960s, the combination of government grants and the income from unregulated hospital insurance offered communities the money to build hospitals, and those hospitals were built more for the community's pride than for its medical needs.

    An example of unnecessary construction costs are the walls required to provide patients rooms with only two beds. Two bed rooms began to appear during the 1960s. Prior to the 1960s, most hospitals had four to six bed rooms for semiprivate patients, and there were ten or more bed wards for charity patients.

    Future hospital construction should build the less expensive to build and maintain four to six bed rooms. In addition to being less expensive to construct, multibed rooms offer patients the opportunity to receive better nursing care. Two bed rooms isolate patients. Nurses must walk up and down long hallways to attend to each patient, and the nurses can not observe their patients. In addition, the communication between nurse and patient is through a public address system.

    Observe the more effective nursing care offered to patients in multibed intensive care areas.

    When asked, my recommendation for hospital construction has been a central core containing the nurse's station, and surrounding the nursing station are a series of four or six bed rooms. The nurses are able to both observe their patients and offer more effective care.

    There will always be patients with illnesses requiring isolation, and they require private rooms. Also, insurance would pay for those rooms; however, the cost of a private room for those individuals not requiring isolation needs to be enough to discourage their use.

2.   Speciality Hospitals.

Another unnecesary hospital fixed cost is the need for all hospitals in a community to offer the same services. Instead, some services need to be restricted to only one community or regional hospital. The cost of providing the equipment and personnel necessary to provide the same service in every community hospital increases the cost of providing the service in each hospital.

Speciality hospitals were common prior to the 1970s, and with the transportation services available today, transferring patients to other hospitals is rarely a problem.

3.   For-profit hospital mangement companies.

Healthcare is not a business, and allowing profits to be obtained from providing hospital services is unconscionable and unprincipled.

I applaud entrepreneurs who establish and profit from business ventures. They are the individuals who have made our country the great nation it has become, and they are the individuals who provide jobs for others. However, healthcare is not the same as a business. (Addendum II)

4.   The cost of a hospital's management.

When the cost of a hospital's management in 1965 is compared with the cost in 2003, the increase is significant, and the increase has had nothing to do with patient care. Those increases have been created by the need for hospitals to comply with unnecessary regulations and documentation requirements and by the excessive salaries and benefits offered to hospital management. Managing a hospital is different than managing business. A hospital would continue to function if its management had made bad decisions; however, a business could be lost if its management had made bad decisions.

For several years as the member of a hospital's Board of Trustees, I was not popular among many of the business persons on the Board during budget discussions. They were unable to understand why I questioned the need for management's salaries and benefits to be so much greater than those offered to nurses. Where were the hospital's priorities? The hospital could not function without nurses, but the hospital could function with a management staff who received less salaries and benefits. Also, why not give the nurses the cars, the country club dues, etc. given to management? Hospital management costs can be reduced by at least 25% to 30%.

5. Hospital regulations.

Hospital regulations and documentation requirements have created significant fixed costs for hospitals, and most of them are unnecessary. They have been created by bureaucratic hospital, government, and HMO administrators who know nothing about medicine. Those regulations and documentation requirements need to be reviewed for their medical necessity by the providers of healthcare's services, and many of them and their costs can be eliminated.

6. Litigation costs.

Hospital litigation costs have become a significant fixed cost, and at least 70% of those costs can be eliminated by endorsing the litigation changes proposed in the fifth change to regulate the private healthcare delivery system.

7. Hospital education programs.

The failure of insurance companies to challenge the cost of a hospital's "education" programs has allowed hospitals to created many unnecessary education programs and to apply their costs as a hospital's fixed cost. Most of those programs contribute nothing towards better patient care, and their funding by a hospitalized patient's insurance needs to be stopped.

An example of an unnecessary education program is a hospital's residency training program. A resident physician is a student, and a patient's hospital insurance should not be subsidizing their education. Allowing those costs to be applied to a hospitalized patient's daily charges should be stopped.

When hospitals had free outpatient clinics and inpatient wards, resident physicians provided those patients their clinical services, and the resident's services were supervised by the hospital's Medical Staff. The residents were paid a small salary for providing those services. In the early 1950s, residents were paid an average of $50 to $75 a month. Unfortunately, unregulated hospital insurance has allowed those salaries to become excessive. At this time, hospitals pay their resident physicians $25,000 to $40,000 annually.

Those salaries are now unnecessary. There are no longer patients in free out-patient clinics or inpatient hospital wards for resident physicians to manage. Instead, residents learn their clinical skills by participating in the management of the hospital's private patients. If private Medical Staff members want the hospital's resident physician to provide their patients services, they should pay the resident for those services.

If a physician wishes to seek speciality training in a hospital, they should expect to do so without funding from a hospitalized patient's insurance. However, if free clinics and inpatient hospital wards appear again, as recommended in one of the six changes, there would be a reason for a hospital's resident physician to receive a salary for their services to those patients, and there would be a reason for insurance to subsidize those salaries. But, the amount of the salary would be much less than those offered at this time.

8.   Marketing programs.

These are an unnecessary fixed cost, and they need to be eliminated. During the 1950s and 1960s, communities constructed hospitals with too many beds, but the hospitals were able to occupy those beds with patients who did not require hospitalization. I can remember during the late 1940s, and during the 1950s, people were admitted to hospitals for their annual physical examinations.

In the 1970s, Medicare initiated a monitoring program to establish the medical necessity of Medicare patients hospital admissions. Many unnecessary admissions were identified, and eliminating those admissions created many empty hospital beds. To attract patients to occupy those beds, hospitals initiated marketing programs.

A hospital's public image should be created by the quality of its services, and not by its marketing program. Also, if hospitals want marketing programs, funding for those programs should no longer be allowed as one of a hospital's fixed costs and paid by hospitalized patient's insurance.

Hospital Variable Costs

Variable costs are those costs created by the services offered to hospitalized patients, and those costs will vary with the number of patients in the hospital and with the cost of the services offered to those patients. A hospital's variable costs can be reduced by:

1. An accounting system to record the cost of the services offered to each hospitalized patient.(DRG's)

2. A penalty for those medical staff members who provide their patients unnecessary services, and

3. Litigation reforms.

Recording the Cost of Patient Services—DRG's:
DRG is an acronym for Diagnostic Related Groups, and the DRGs should be used to account for the cost of the services each patient receives.

When Medicare was initiated, hospitals were unable to tell Medicare the cost of treating different diseases and disorders. The faculty at Yale University developed an accounting system for Medicare. It classified all diseases, disorders and procedures into 473 DRGs. When a Medicare patient is discharged from a hospital, their disorder, disease, or procedure is assigned a DRG, and all of the services the patient received during their hospitalization as well as their costs were recorded in the patient's DRG.

DRGs offer three pieces of valuable information about a hospital's variable costs.

1. DRGs identify the cost of treating different diseases or disorders in every community and regional hospital.

2. DRGs compare the cost of treating the same disease or disorder in different hospitals, and

3. DRGs enable hospitals to compare the cost of the services offered by different Medical Staff members treating the same diseases or disorders.

Applying the DRGs to account for each patient's services makes each Medical Staff member accountable for the cost of the services they offer their patients.

Penalties for Unnecessary Services:
The second way to reduce a hospital's variable costs is to have a financial penalty for staff members who offer unnecesary services. A bed tax is an appropriate penalty. When a patient is admitted to the hospital, the patient's physician is charged a daily "tax" for each day the patient is hospitalized. If the cost of the services offered a patient during their hospitalization is equal to, or less than, the average DRG cost for treating the same disease or disorder in the region, the physician (Medical Staff member) does not have to pay the hospital's bed tax for that patient.

The bed tax must be large enough to have Medical Staff members consider seriously the medical necessity of the services they offer their patients.

Hospital litigation:
Will the public ever recognize how litigation is increasing the cost of everything they purchase? This is especially true in healthcare. Litigation is the major cause of the increasing cost of a hospital's variable costs. Neither the DRGs nor the bed tax will contribute to reducing a hospital's variable costs unless there is litigation reform. The out-of-control litigation system in the United States forces every hospital's Medical Staff member to provide their patients many unnecessary services to protect themseves if their patient initiates a lawsuit. The physician wants to have every possible test on the patient's chart prior to the lawsuit. Furthermore, no physician will be willing to monitor the medical necessity of the services of another physician until there is litigation protection.

Resistance to the proposed changes in a hospital's allowable fixed cost can be expected from the business oriented multihospital management companies. Many, if not most, hospitals have become multihospital business systems, and they are profit driven with investors. Suggesting programs to reduce their revenues will be challenged. Likewise, resistance can be expected from some physicians to changing a hospital's allowable fixed costs and to using the DRGs to account for variable costs. Many hospital services such as Outpatient Surgical Centers and some hospitals are physician owned. Reducing their revenues will not be popular.

If only the public could learn, they benefit from reducing hospital costs. In contrast, the multihospital managemenrt companies do not benefit nor do the physician owned hospitals and hospital serevices. Will the public become more politically active and achieve what benefits them? Or, will the multihospital management companies and some entrepreneural physicians achieve what benefits them? The public has the advantage. They have the power of their vote. Who is going to be the winner?

11

Litigation Reform.

Litigation reform is the fifth change to regulate a private healthcare delivery system.

There is no challenge to this statement! The most serious threat to the quality and availability of the public's future healthcare services is the out-of-control litigation system in the United States. No other country exposes its physicians or its businesses to such abusive litigation.

Litigation reform is necessary regardless of whether the public's healthcare services are delivered by a private delivery system, by a National Health Service, or by the HMO industry. Without litigation reform, the healthcare delivery system along with the manufacturing segment of our economy will collapse in the next decade. Signs of their collapse are visible already. As has been identified, a delivery system is only as good as the physicians who provide its services. At this time, fewer physicians are willing to accept patients requiring "high risk" services such as emergency room services, neurosurgical services, complicated pregnancies, and the problems associated with early births. Also, over the past decade, the harrassment of physicians by irresponsibly initiated malpractice lawsuits and the cost of protecting themselves from such lawsuits has contributed to an increasing number of physicians who are no longer interested in remaining in, or encouraging others to enter, healthcare.

In addition, the increasing number of the higher paying manufacturing jobs leaving the country are signs the manufacturing segment of our economy is beginning to collapse. The business community is tired of the increasing cost of product liability insurance; is tired of the increasing cost of defending themselves against irresponsibly initiated product liability lawsuits; is tired of the increasing number of employee initiated lawsuits; and is tired of the increasing dollar amounts of jury awards. To escape from those escalating litigation costs, the busi-

51

ness community is actively seeking technology to replace their emloyees, and is actively seeking manufacturing opportunites outside of the United States.

Many individuals mistakenly believe jobs are leaving the United States because of labor costs. Apparently, they are wrong. Labor costs are a problem for many manufacturers, but studies have shown labor costs are not the primary reason many of those jobs are leaving the United States. Otherwise, Europe and Japan would not be obtaining many of those jobs. Both European countries and Japan have relatively high labor costs. However, they have low healthcare costs (6–9% of their GNPs), they do not have antibusiness litigation problems, and they do not have the large business taxes they are required to pay in the United States. All of these lower costs are attractive to businesses.

Few among the public appear to realize how both the medical community and the business community are tired of being harrassed by many irresponsibly initiated lawsuits. If the public is serious about maintaining a quality healthcare delivery system in the United States as well as retaining more employment opportunities, they had best give some serious thought to the importance of their role in changing the litigation process in our country. Unfortunately, there is no evidence the public is interest in, or is willing to participate in, litigation reform. The public has failed to support the medical community's attempts to obtain relief from malpractice litigation costs, and the public has failed to understand how abusive litigation along with increasing employee health benefit costs and taxes are forcing businesses to leave the United States along with their jobs.

Malpractice lawsuits were not a problem prior to the1960s. Prior to the 1960s, the patient's pocketbook was the primary source of payment for healthcare's services, and healthcare had no "deep pockets". However, during the 1960s and 1970s, money from unregulated health insurance programs began to flow into the healthcare delivery system, and healthcare acquired "deep pockets". Those "deep pockets" attracted attorneys, and the number of malpractice lawsuits increased. At this time, malpractice litigation is estimated to cost the healthcare delivery system at least 50 billion dollars each year, and those billions of litigation costs do not include the billions of additional dollars required to pay for the many unnecessary services physicians are forced to offer their patients to protect themselves from frivolous lawsuits. Instead of purchasing healthcare services for patients, those billions of healthcare's dollars are providing attorneys generous incomes.

Litigation was one the four reasons offered previously as the major causes for increasing healthcare costs, and litigation has caused the increasing costs of the other three. For example, the threat of litigation has created the need for providers to offer their patients unnecessary services; the cost of litigation has increased the cost of malpractice insurance; and the cost of malpractice insurance has required providers to increase their fees. In addition, litigation has increased the costs associated with the need for providers to comply with the many unnecessary regulations and documentation requirements.

An example of the cost of our abusive litigation system in the United States is the lawsuit I experienced as a member of a hospital's Board of Trustees. A patient was suing a member of the hospital's medical staff. Because the hospital had approved the physician's credentials, the hospital was included in the patient's lawsuit. In addition, since the Board of Trustees had approved the hospital's approval of the physician's credentials, each member of the Board of Trustees was included in the lawsuit. The lawsuit was frivolous, but the cost of defending the physician, the hospital, and each member of the Board of Trustees was enormous.

The public's complacency about litigation reform has both the business and healthcare communities captives of an out-of-control litigation system. Wake up America!!! It will require the power of your vote to change the litigation system in the United States. Have you given no thought to your future, or to your family's future, healthcare services or to your future employment opportunities? You are asked to think one more time about who will be providing your healthcare services in the next decade. Attorneys can not provide those services. And, remember training a physician requires more than a decade. If the public is disatisfied with their physicians as well as their numbers in the next decade, it will require another decade to train more physicians. The public will have two decades to live with their physician concerns.

Since malpractice litigation has become such a profitable business for the legal profession, litigation reform will NOT be accomplished by either the medical or the business communities. The attorney dominated State legislatures will never initiate realistic litigation reforms without the pressure of the public's vote. Legislators want to be reelected, and because of their wish to be reelected, an informed and politically active public can easily achieve litigation reforms favorable to themselves. Yes, there is a powerful trial lawyers lobby contributing much money to oppose any change in the existing litigation process, but the public has the advantage. It is their vote. Once the public becomes aware of the negative long range consequences of no litigation reform, they will write, telephone, and email their elected representatives in both state legislatures and in Congress demanding the litigaton reforms they want to be enacted into law. Otherwise, those representatives can not expect the public's vote at the next election.

The proposed litigation reforms offer the public the oppportunity to offer their elected representatives litigation reforms they can enact into law.

Before discussing the proposed litigation reforms, four major problems with the existing malpractice litigation system need to be identified and discussed. Understanding them is necessary to understanding the proposed reforms.

Those four problems are:

1.   The cost of defense.

2.   The absence of responsibility and accountability.

3.   The jury system.

4.   The court system tolerating frivolous lawsuits.

1. The cost of defense:
Defending physicians in malpractice lawsuits has become a "cash cow" for trial lawyers and an enormous expense for physicians and hospitals. Every malpractice lawsuit requires an attorney be employed regardless of whether the physician or hospital is guilty or innocent. The cost of employing attorneys to defend physicians and hospitals against many frivolous malpractice lawsuits is the major cause of escalating malpractice insurance costs.

Some individuals have claimed the increasing cost of malpractice insurance has been caused by large jury awards, and placing a "cap" on jury awards has been suggested. Although jury awards contribute to the cost of litigation, they are not a significant cost problem. Others have suggested insurance company mismanagement and provider incompetency have been the major cause of escalating malpractice insurance costs. However, neither jury awards, insurance company mismanagement, nor provider incompetency have been the major causes for the escalating cost of malpractice insurance. The primary cause of those increasing costs has been, and remains, the cost of defense. It is the need for insurance companies to employ many attorneys to defend their insured physicians and hospitals against the flood of frivolous malpractice lawsuits in the United States.

During the 1980s, I participated in the review of malpractice lawsuits, and approximately 80% of malpractice lawsuits were judged to have no malpractice during either a deposition or jury trial. However, the expense of employing attorneys to defend those physicians in those depositions and jury trials was enormous. For example, at the time, approximately 60 cents of every dollar a physician paid for their malpractice insurance was paid to those attorneys employed by the insurance companies to defend them. Employing attorneys and paying for the other costs generated by attorneys was the major cost for malpractice insurance companies in the 1980s, and I understand the numbers are the same in 2002.

Someone has applied the word "maloccurence" to malpractice litigation, and it is important for the public to understand its meaning. It explains why so many "frivolous" lawsuits (no malpractice) are initiated, and it explains why the cost of employing attorneys to defend against those frivolous lawsuits has become the major cause of escalating malpractice insurance costs.

What is "malocurrence"? Any recommended treatment program may have an unsatisfactory outcome. If a physician or hospital error is the cause of the unsatisfactory outcome, the problem is "malpractice". However, if the physician or hospital did everything properly and the outcome was unsatisfactory, the problem is "maloccurrence". Asking a jury selected from among the general population to make the judgement between malpractice and maloccurrence is not reasonable and is no longer acceptable. Special courts are needed to hear malpractice lawsuits.

Maloccurrence, or a bad outcome, can happen in spite of everything being done to prevent an unsatisfactory outcome, and the cost of defending against maloccurence lawsuits creates an enormous unnecessary cost problem. When I was reviewing malpractice lawsuits, I would find about two or possibly three out of every ten lawsuits I reviewed to have malpractice. The other seven or eight were maloccurrence. Nevertheless, those maloccurrence lawsuits required the cost of employing attorneys to defend them. The only way to eliminate the unnecessary cost of defending against maloccurrence lawsuits is to endorse the "loser pays all" policy to be described in the recommended litigation reforms.

2. The second problem with the existing litigation system is the absence of any responsibility for having initiated a frivolous lawsuit and the absence of any financial accountability for the costs a lawsuit has created for those being sued. The absence of both responsibility and financial accountability are the reasons so many maloccurrence lawsuits are initiated. Initiating lawsuits in the United States has become a lottery. Initiate a lawsuit an hope you win. It will cost you nothing.

3. The third major problem with litigation is the jury system. An individual is supposed to be judged by a jury of their peers. The present selection of jurers from among the general population does not offer a physician the opportunity to be judged by a jury of his, or her's, peers. Jurers selected from among the general population do not possess the knowledge necessary to make an informed judgement about the medical issues in a malpractice lawsuit. Furthermore, the use of an "expert witness" to inform a jury about the medical issues in a lawsuit does not provide a jury unbiased information. Expert witnesses are employed by attorneys, and they function as "hired guns" for the attorneys who have employed them. Also, most expert witnesses are not trained in court room procedures, and their testimonies are frequently and easily discredited by attorneys during crossexaminations.

The increasing complexity of the healthcare issues requires special malpractice courts be established, similiar to the bankruptcy courts, to replace the selection of jury members from among the general population.

4. The fourth problem with the litigation system is a court system tolerating frivolous lawsuits. To justify those lawsuits, the court's defense is, "The public is entitled to their day in court". I would agree, every individual is entitled to there day in court; however, when an individual uses that day, they have the responsibility of initiating a valid lawsuit and if they lose their lawsuit, they should be accountable for any costs created by their lawsuit.

The public is encouraged to endorse the following proposed litigation reforms, and to use the power of their vote to have their elected representatives enact them into law. Remember, it is your future healthcare delivery system—and your jobs. To think about a healthcare delivery system and a business community without litigation reform should be frightening to everyone.

The proposed litigation reforms are:

1. An attorney's contingency fee would be retained.

2. All local Medical and Osteopathic Societies will establish a Malpractice Review Committee. Once a malpractice lawsuit is intiated, the insurance company will refer the lawsuit to a Society's Malpractice Review Committee in an area where the physician being sued does not practice. The Committee will appoint at least two providers from the community to a Malpractice Review Team. The Team members will provide the same service as the one contained in the lawsuit.

The Team's review of the lawsuit offers the physician being sued the opportunity to be judged by a jury of his, or her's, peers. Also, if the lawsuit goes to a jury trial, the Team can provide the jury members more objective information about the medical issues in the lawsuit than can an "expert witness" employed by either attorney.

Jurers have problems understanding the conflicting testimony of different "expert witnesses". I have listened to physicians employed as "experts" make erroneous statements during their testimony. When their statements were challenged by another physician, the jury members did not possess the knowledge necessary to understand the difference in the two physician's statements. As a result, the jury's decision became more of an emotional decision rather than an informed decision.

Objections to a Society's Team members reviewing malpractice lawsuits have been offered. Those objections focus on the Team members bias. The Team members would attempt to protect the physician being sued. This is paranoia! Nothing could be further from the truth. Malpractice lawsuits have been objectively reviewed by many physicians. In my experience, when two physicians are asked to review the same ten lawsuits, both would agreed the same two or possibly three of the ten lawsuits had malpractice. The use of Team members to evaluate malpractice lawsuits is far superior to the present use of physicians employed by attorneys as expert witnesses. Furthermore, the team members evaluating the merits of a lawsuit will be from communities other than the one in which the physician being sued practices.

Team members will be reimbursed by the insurance company requesting the review, and the reimbursement will be based on the Provider Reimbursement Formula. All community providers will be required to accept an assignment to their local Society's Malpractice Review Teams regardless of whether or not they are members of their local Society. The penalty could be the refusal of the malpractice insurancce company to offer the physician coverage in the future.

3. The Team's review of the lawsuit is referred back to the Society's Malpractice Review Committee, and the Committee sends the Team's report to both attorneys.

4. Both attorneys, as well as their "expert witnesses", have the opportunity to question and crossexamine the Team's members during a deposition.

5. If the lawsuit goes as far as a trial, my preference is to have the selection of jury members from the general population replaced by a special malpractice court and to have the Team members testify in that court environment. There are speciality courts for other special legal issues, and there is no reason why a malpractice lawsuit should not be presented in a special court.

If the trial is to be by a jury selected from among the general population, the Team members would present their findings to the jury, and only the members of the jury and the judge, if necesssary, can question the Team's members. Team members will not be subjected to a crossexamination by either attorney in front of the jury. The attorneys and their expert witnesses had their opportunity to crossexamine the Team's members during the deposition.

Following over ten years of providing testimony during several jury trials, my observation has been the crossexamination of a witness by an attorney in front of a jury is primarily to discredit the witness and confuse the jury rather than to inform the jury. As I learned several times during crossexaminations, discrediting a physician is not a difficult task for an experienced trial attorney. I am aware of two lawsuits I believe I lost for patients during my crossexaminations, and both patients had valid lawsuits. Physicians, like myself, are not trained in court room procedures or crossexamination techniques, and we are easily confused.

To illustrate how easily a physician's testimony can be discredited, an attorney said to me following several hours of testimony, "Doctor, how many grafts have you taken from the area in question? I said, "Several." He said in a loud voice, "Doctor, you testified you had never taken grafts from the area." During my deposition one year previously I had said, "I have never taken grafts of this size from the area." The attorney had neglected to include my statement "of this size" in his question to me. My attempts to quickly review the many pages of my deposition taken the previous year to discover what I had said, made me appear confused, and I am confident the attorney had successfully discredited me in the minds of the jury.

6. The "loser pays all" policy.
The "loser pays all" policy is a must if the costs associated with malpractice litgation are to be reduced. The "loser pays all" policy states you have the right to initiate a lawsuit; however, if you lose your lawsuit, you will pay the defense costs of those you have sued.

At this time, the individual initiating a lawsuit has no expenses. It costs them nothing to initiate a lawsuit, and they will have had no expenses if they lose their lawsuit. But, the individual being sued has had the expense of employing an attorney to defend themselves, as well as other defense costs, and if they successfully defend themselves, they have no way of recovering any of their attorney's fees or other defense costs.

The "loser pays all" policy restores responsibility to litigation. If an individual knows they may have to pay the defense expenses of those they have sued, they will be more responsible about initiating their lawsuit, and my estimate is at least 70% of present lawsuits would never be initiated. Or, about 70% of existing litigation costs will be eliminated.

Obtaining public support for the "loser pays all" may not be easy. Aside from the public's complacency about litigation issues, many individuals are misinformed. They believe a "loser pays all" policy would threaten their Constitutional "right" to initiate a lawsuit. It does not. It only requires them to be responsible for their lawsuit and accountable for its financial damages.

Obtaining a "loser pays all" policy may require a constitutional amendment in some states instead of their legislatures enacting the policy into law. However, the public should not fear the need for a constitutional amendment. It would receive the support of an informed and politically active public. If states like Florida can have their voters pass a no smoking in restaurants amendment, a "loser pays all" could be passed as well.

Perhaps the public's major challenge to obtaining a "loser pays all" policy is the legal profession's loss of income. The policy will require fewer attorneys to initiate, as well as to defend against, malpractice lawsuits, and attorneys can not be expected to accept this loss of income quietly. Their trial lawyer's lobby will actively oppose the "loser pays all" policy. Imagine the lost income for attorneys if 70% of present lawsuits are never initiated.

In addition to significantly reducing the number of malpractice lawsuits and their costs, the "loser pays all" policy offers the public a better opportunity to win valid lawsuits. I have witnessed several patients with valid malpractice lawsuits lose their lawsuits. Why? Attorneys know jurys are sympathethic towards physicians. Accordingly, attorneys ecourage physicians guilty of malpractice to seek jury trials, and many of those physicians receive favorable jury decisions. However, if there was a "loser pays all" policy, fewer physicians guilty of malpractice would be requesting jury trials in the hope of acquiring a favorable jury decision.

For example, if a Society's Team members had identified malpractice, and if the Team would be presenting their decision to a jury without an attorney's crossexamination, the physician would realize the odds were against a jury finding them not guilty of malpractice. Also, the physician would realize they, and not their insurance company, would have to pay for the costs of the trial. Accordingly, rather than initiating a jury trial in the hope of obtainig a favorable jury decision, the physician guilty of malpractice would settled the lawsuit with their patient.

Litigation has become an extremely profitable business for attorneys, and the public is going to be overwhelmed with misinformation from those who seek to maintain the existing litigation system. As the public ponders the importance of litigation reform to themselves and to their families, they need to keep in mind the physician holds the key to the quality of the healthcare services offered by a healthcare delivery system. If the present litigation system remains, there will be fewer individuals attracted to healthcare to become future physicians, and many of those who become physicians will not have come from the best of our youth.

12

Litigation Reform and The Public's Indifference.

What is the public's problem? Why they have they failed to support their physician's legislative efforts to achieve realistic malpractice reforms? The public's indifference to malpractice reform, and to other litigation reforms, has to be a concern for every person in the United States. Their future healthcare delivery system, as well as their jobs, depends on the public's use of their vote to force litigation reforms. Without it, both will collapse within a decade. The public is reminded, physicians provide their healthcare services, and manufacturing companies provide them higher paying jobs. Abusive litigation is forcing too many physicians to leave medicine and to discourage others from entering medicine, and it is forcing too many manufacturers to leave the country with their jobs.

Perhaps some among the public believe the existing litigation system does not effect them. They are so wrong! Every provider's service and every manufacturer's product has a significant litigation cost attached to its price. For example, in the early 1950s, the cost of my malpractice insurance was only a few hundred dollars. However, when I retired in1990, the cost of my malpractice insurance had increased to several thousand dollars. Those increased insurance costs were paid by my patients. My fees had to be increased to pay for those costs.

The litigation costs attached to every service and product is paid by the public, and it is the public who is providing attorneys the incomes required to pay for their expensive advertisements on billboards, on TV, and on radio. Yes, the existing litigation system does effect the public. It is costing them billions of dollars unnecessarily.

Some individuals may believe the existing litigation system benefits them. They believe if the existing litigation system were changed, they would not be able to afford to engage the attorneys of their choice to initiate their lawsuits. This is so wrong. The recommended litigation reforms continue to provide attorneys the opportuity to offer their clients contingency fees. Their clients can engage their services without a fee, and the attorney will be paid a percentage of any awards.

Some individuals may believe the cost of lawsuits is a problem for insurance companies and not for themselves. This is so wrong. Yes, insurance companies pay for the defense against most lawsuits, and they pay the cost of jury awards and other lawsuit settlements; however, the money the insurance companies use to pay those costs is the public's money. The only money insurance companies have is the money they collect from the public when the public pays their insurance premiums.

The following is an example of how frivolous litigation is contributing to the increasing cost of the public's automobile insurance. To paraphrase what an orthopedic surgeon said to me several years ago, "An attorney's letter to an insurance company for a client claiming a whiplash neck or back injury from a minor auto accident is worth about $5,000 or more." Yes, insurance companies are willing to settle a frivolous claim for that amount of money to prevent the expense of future litigation. When you consider the attorney collects about 30% or more of the insurance company's settlement with their client, the attorney makes an easy profit of $1,500 or more from each letter. I imagine orthopedic surgeons are experiencing the same problem today. And, the public continues to complain about their rising automobile insurance costs. They need to realize they are the problem!

Is the public aware of employers who are forced to discharge employees rather than have to face a lawsuit. There are numerous examples of employers discharging employees to prevent having to defend themselves against a frivlously initiated sex discrimination lawsuit. Yes, the employer would probably win such a lawsuit, but the cost of defending themselves is too much. It is less expensive to fire the employee. Yes, a frivolously initiated sex discrimination lawsuit could result in the loss of your job.

Hopefully, the public will become aware of how serious the litigation problem has become in our country, and they will be motivated to offer their support for the recommended litigation reforms. The power of their vote offers the public the opportunity to obtain any legislation they want. Will, they use it to reform litigation?

13

Establishing Free Outpatient and Inpatient Facilities.

The sixth proposed change to regulate a private healthcare delivery system is to establish free outpatient and inpatient healthcare facilities like those that existed prior to the 1970s.

For many years before the introduction of health and hospital insurance, large cities and all communities had hospitals providing free healthcare services in outpatient clinics an in inpatient hospital wards. Also, individuals entering medicine expected to provide, and did provide, free services to patients unable to pay for them in those free hospital facilities. as well as in their offices. The gifts patients offered my wife and me in payment for my services back in the 1950s were special.

In the early 1970s, insurance had become the primary source of payment for healthcare's services, and most patients no longer required free services. The free clinics and hospital wards began to close. However, there continued to be patients without insurance and without the ability to pay for their services, and they were having, and continue to have, difficulty obtaining their necessary services.

Health and hospital insurance will continue to provide most individuals the opportunity to pay for their healthcare services, but there will always be individuals who will be unable to pay for those services for whatever reason. Those individuals will require a healthcare delivery system to provide them free services as they were provided prior to the 1970s. And, like prior to the 1970s, those free services can be provided by a regulated private healthcare delivery system.

The free facilities would be located in most hospitals, as they were prior to the 1970s, and staffing those free facilities would not be a problem. Hospitals offer their medical staff members special opportunities. They can practice their profession and generate incomes while using the hospital's equipment, personnel, and other resources at no cost to themselves. Prior to the 1970s, in return for the opportunity to admit patients to the hospital and to use the hospital's resources, Medical Staff members were obligated to participate in the treatment of patients in their hospital's free inpatient wards and outpatient clinics. The practice should be continued.

In addition to a hospital's Medical Staff members participating in their hospital's free outpatient clinics, other physicians will be eager to participate in those outpatient facilities. It provides them the opportunity to maintain their clinical skills by treating patients who have diseases and disorders they may not see in their offices. This was the practice prior to the closing of those free facilities, and it should be continued.

Funding for the space, for the nursing staffs, and for the other administrative expenses could become an allowable fixed cost for a hospital, and those costs could be applied to each hospitalized patient's daily charges and paid by their insuarance.

The free facilities could become part of a hospital's Department of Family Practice and the facilities incorporated into the emergency room's space.

14

Seeking Additional Legislative Support For The Six Changes.

When, and if, the public decides it is to their advantage to support the six changes to regulate a private healthcare delivery system, they should seek the support of Medical and Osteopathic Societies; seek the support of the business community; seek the support of labor unions; and seek the support of the private health insurance industry. All will benefit from the proposed six changes.

The members of Medical and Osteopathic Societies would benefit by having:

a.   the opportunity to be independent practitioners in a fee-for-service private healthcare delivery system rather than be an employee of a National Health Service or an employee of a managed healthcare company (HMO).

b.   the opportunity to receive reimbursements for their services established by the Provider Reimbursement Formula rather than arbitarily established by a third party.

c.   the opportunity to have ALL healthcare dollars spent purchasing healthcare services rather than spent supporting the salaries, benefits, and operating costs of another government bureaucracy or of a managed healthcare company.

d.   the opportunity to treat patients who have had the freedom to select the providers of their choice.

e.   the opportunity to determine their patient's needs, independent of a third party's approval.

f.   the opportunity to have the medical necessity of their services challenged by peers who possess the appropriate qualifications to make those challenges.

g.   the opportunity to offer their patients more comprehensive, better quality, and more easily available services, at a lower cost than those offered by either an HMO or a National Health Service,

h.   the opportunity to have the cost of their malpractice insurance reduced significantly,

i.   the opportunity to stop offering their patients unnecessary services to protect themselves from frivolous lawsuits, and

j.   the opportunity to review and eliminate many of the administratively expensive and unnecessary regulations and documentation requirements established by HMOs and government.

The Business Comminity.
The business community will benefit by having the cost of their employee's healthcare benefits reduced by at least 40% within five years; will benefit by preserving for themselves, for their families, and for their employees the many patient benefits offered by a private healthcare delivery system; will benefit by avoiding the taxes required to support a National Health Service; will benefit by having their litigation costs reduced significantly; and will benefit by having the cost of the goods and services they purchase to operate their businesses reduced as their supplier's health benefits and litigation costs are reduced, as well as their taxes.

Labor Unions.
The reduction in every employer's healthcare and litigation costs, as well as their taxes, will benefit labor unions. Those reductions will encourage employers to retain the better paying manufacturing jobs in the United States, and those reductions will enable the cost of their manufactured products to remain competitive in the international marketplace. Another benefit for labor unions would be the absence of the personal income taxes their members would be required to pay to support a National Health Service. Paying fewer taxes provides their members more money in their pockets to spend purchasing "things". Those additional purchases require manufacturers to produce more "things", and producing more "things" requires more people be employed to manufacture those additional "things". In addition, reducing the healthcare and litigation costs, as well as the

business taxes required to support a National Health Service, offers manufacturers the opportunity to offer union members the opportunity to purchase all of their "things" less expensively.

The Insurance Industry.
The reductions in the cost of healthcare's services will reduce the cost of an indemnity insurance company's premiums significantly, and without the management, the operating, the investor, and the other expenses of the HMO industry, the indemnity insurance industry's premiums would become less expensive than those offered by the HMO industry. (Addendum III)

15

A Message To Congress.

Most of the people with whom I have spoken are not aware of, nor do they feel threatened by, the long range consequences of a National Health Service whose services are offered by a profit driven managed healthcare company (HMO). As a result, they have not considered their need to preserve a private healthcare delivery system. Hopefully, this book will start the public thinking about their need to preserve a private healthcare delivery system, and motivate them to become the political activists necessary to preserve the system.

When, and if, the public becomes aware of their need to preserve the private healthcare delivery system, and when, and if, it is not too late, their message to Congress should be:

1. the ONLY two problems with the existing private healthcare delivery system are the cost of its services and its failure to provide easily available services to those individuals without insurance or without the ability to pay for their services, and

2. the ONLY cause of those two problems has been, and continues to be, the patient and the provider abuses of unregulated health and hospital insurance programs, and

3. those insurance abuses can be overcome by adopting six changes to regulate the existing private healthcare delivery system, and

4. those six changes will provide the necessary reductions in healthcare's costs and have those costs become internationally competitive (8% to 9% of the GNP), and

5. neither the cost of the bureaucracy necessary to administer a National Health Service nor the cost of the management and operating expenses necessary to

maintain the HMO industry will allow either to achieve the reductions in healthcare's costs that are possible by endorsing the proposed six changes to regulate the existing private healthcare delivery system, and

6. neither a National Health Service nor the HMO industry can offer the public quality, comprehensive, and easily available services as inexpensively as those offered by a private delivery system whose costs and service utilization are regulated by the proposed six changes in the existing private healthcare delivery system, and

7. although both a National Health Service and the HMO industry can offer the public their healthcare services, only physicians and other healthcare professionals can provide those services, and

8. neither Medicare (government) nor the HMO industry have offered, nor do they possess the ability to offer, the career incentives necessary to attract the best from among our youth into healthcare to become the providers of the public's future healthcare services, and

9. we, the public, want to maintain a private healthcare delivery system, and to achieve that goal, we want six changes to regulate a private healthcare delivery system to become the law. And, we will use our vote to insure the six changes are adopted and a private healthcare delivery system preserved. All of the material necessary to implement the proposed six changes exists, and they can be organized into a structured program by a small staff within months.

The importance of the public using the power of their vote to insure Congress maintains a private healthcare delivery system can not be overemphasized. Its advantages have been discussed. As the public ponders the value of their challenging government's attempts to replace the private healthcare delivery system with one they can control, the public should consider the following:

1. Do I want to allow government to do to the healthcare delivery system what it has done to the education system in the United States? We have the most expensive and the worst education system in the industrialized world.

2. Can government provide my healthcare services? No, it can only offer those services. Physicians provide them.

3. If government only offers my healthcare services, can I be sure of the quality and the availability of those services? No! Their quality and availablity depends on the physicians providing them.

4. If the quality and the availability of my healthcare services depends on the physicians providing them, would I want to spend ten to fifteen years of my life studying to be a physician whose future is an employee of a National Health Service or of an HMO? Of course not.

Addendum I

Healthcare and Price Controls

The Provider Reimbursement Formula introduces price controls. Are they necessary? Yes, and physicians are ecouraged to endorse them. Why? Since health and hospital insurance will continue to be the primary source of payment for healthcare's services, and since insurance will continue to insulated the public from their need to consider the cost of those services, price controls have become necessary.

There are valid arguments against price controls effectively controlling prices in a free market economy. But, the healthcare delivery system is not a free market economy. In a free market economy, the consumer has the option of deciding whether or not they want to purchase a service, and the consumer's purchases determine the demand for, the supply of, as well as the price of those services. In contrast, the consumer (patient) in the healthcare delivery system does not have the option of deciding whether or not they want to purchase a medically necessary service. The consumer (patient) must receive the service. Furthermore, unlike the free market economy, the patient's purchases of healthcare's services do not determine the demand for, the supply of, or the price of, those service. Instead, healthcare's providers create the demand for, the supply of, and the price of healthcare's services.

One example of how providers create the demand for, and establish the price of, healthcare's services is the government's unsuccessful attempt to reduce the cost of healthcare's services by encouraging competition among providers by increaing their numbers. The government subsidized the expansion of medical school classes to enable them to graduate more physicians, and many foreign trained physicians were encouraged to entered the United States; however, as their numbers increased so did healthcare's costs. Why? Those additional physicians were able to create the demand for additional services. They were able to offer their Medicare patients additional services unchallenged, and many of those services were unnecessary. Furthermore, those additional physicians were able to establish the price (their charges) for those services unchallenged. A fact: as long as providers have the ability to create the demand for, and establish the price of, healthcare's services, creating competiton among providers to reduce healthcare's costs is meaningless.

Another example of how providers have been able to establish the demand for healthcare's services was the government's attempts to introduce price controls. The payments for Medicare's services were frozen. However, healthcare's costs continued to increase. Why? Again, providers were able to offer their Medicare patients additional services to compensate for their frozen reimbursements.

These examples illustrate why the only way to reduce and stabilize healthcare's costs is to have both price controls and monitoring for the medical necessity of the services patients receive. Price controls stabilize the price of a service and monitoring for medical necessity establishes the medical necessity of the service and prevents unnecesary services from being offered to compensate for the price controls. (Monitoring was discussed as the third change to regulate the private healthcare delivery system).

Healthcare price controls are not new. Both Medicare and the manage healthcare industry (HMOs) have unsuccessfully applied price controls for the past two decades. In addition to their failure to control the cost of healthcare's services, those price controls have failed to offer providers career incentives, and the absence of career incentives has demoralized too many physicians and other healthcare providers. Another problem is the failure of either Medicare or the HMO industry to apply price controls to themselves. They applied price controls to their provider's fees, but they applied no controls on the amount of healthcare's dollars they could spend to support the increasing costs of the expanding Medicare bureaucracy and the increasing costs of the managed healthcare industry's management and operating expenses.

Price controls are necessary, but price controls must offer physicians and other healthcare providers career incentives. Without career incentives, price controls will threaten both the quality and the availability of the public's future healthcare services. The best from among our country's youth will no longer be attacted to medicine. Another reminder: there is a significant difference between a delivery system offering the public their healthcare services and physicians providing those services. This fact can not be overemphasized. To encourage the best from among our country's youth to become physicians, career incentives must be offered to them.

The price controls proposed in the six changes to regulate the existing private delivery system offer physicians career incentives. They are:

a.   the opportunity to be independent practitioners in a fee-for-service private healthcare delivery system rather than an employee of either a National Health Service or a managed healthcare company (HMO).

b.   the opportunity to receive reimbursements for their services established by the Provider Reimbursement Formula rather than arbitarily established by a third party.

c.   the opportunity to have ALL healthcare dollars spent on purchasing health-care services rather than supporting the salaries and operational costs of another government bureaucracy or of a managed healthcare company.

d.   the opportunity to treat patients who have had the freedom to select the pro-viders of their choice,

e.   the opportunity to determine their patient's needs, independent of a third party's approval.

f.   the opportunity to have the challenges to the medical necessity of their ser-vices made by peers whose qualifications to make those challenges are appro-priate.

g.   the opportunity to have the cost of their malpractice insurance reduced sig-nificantly.

h.   the opportunity to offer their patients more comprehensive, better quality, and more easily available services, at a lower cost than those offered by either an HMO or a National Health Service, and

i.   The opportunity to stop having the need to offer their patients unnecessary services to protect themselves from frivolous lawsuits.

The Provider Reimbursement Formula's price controls offer physicians both career incentives and an acceptable method of calculating their reimbursements. In addition, the six changes to regulate a private delivery system provide the medical necessity monitoring required to support the price controls, and they return the responsibility for medical necessity monitoring to local Medical and Osteopathic Societies where it belongs.

Addendum II

Healthcare is not a Business.

During the 1970s, the easy profits from unregulated health and hospital insurance attracted businesspersons with their investors. Together, they created the managed healthcare industry (HMOs and multihospital companies), and over two decades, they transformed the practice of medicine into the healthcare delivery system. As discussed previously, the practice of medicine was a profession dedicated to providing healthcare services to all in need of those services, regardless of their ability to pay. In contrast, the healthcare delivery system is a business driven delivery system dedicated to generating profits from the sale of healthcare's services to only those who can afford to purchase them.

Over the past thirty years, the managed healthcare industry has attempted to demonstrate its ability to control healthcare's costs by "managing" the delivery of healthcare's services. But, they have failed, and the industry has made obtaining necessary services increasingly difficult for those individuals unable to pay for their services. In addition, the industry's salaries, benefits, and other personnel costs, along with their other operating, administrative, and investor expenses, are consuming many healthcare dollars that would be better spent purchasing healthcare services for patients.

The reason the managed healthcare companies have failed, and will continue to fail, is healthcare is different than a business system. The following are a few of the differences.

A successful business has an operating budget. However, the variable costs associated with the variety of services required to diagnose and to treat the many different diseases and disorders make projecting those variable costs into a budget extremely difficult, if not impossible. Also, the attempts to control those variable costs by approving the services recommended by physicians prior to the patient receiving those services has been a failure. Many patients have been denied necessary services unnecessarily, and their treatment has been compromised. The "management" of healthcare's variable costs is best accomplished by physicians, and the six changes to regulate a private delivery system offer physicians the appropriate tools to manage those variable costs.

A business has a management team who designs a business plan and who directs the company's resources to achieve the goals of the business plan. In contrast, healthcare has the physician who designs the treatment plan and who directs the application of healthcare's resources to achieve the goals of the treatment plan.

There is a difference between the business and healthcare consumer. The business consumer has three options. First, they have the option of deciding if they want to purchase the business service. Second, they have the option of deciding the price they are willing to pay for the service. Third, they have the option of going to different providers seeking a better price for the same service, and they can be assured the quality of that service will be the same at all of the different providers. For example, the quality of the same model new automobile is the same at all the dealerships.

In contrast, the healthcare consumer has neither the option of deciding if they want to purchase a necesssary healthcare service nor the option of deciding the price they are willing to pay for the service. They must have the service, and they must pay whatever is necessary to acquire it. Furthermore, although the healthcare consumer has the option of going to different providers seeking a better price for the same service, they can not be assured the quality of the same service offered by different providers will be the same. There are doctors, and there are doctor's doctors. The doctor's doctor is the doctor whose services are recognized as being superior by other doctors and whose services other doctors seek for themselves and for their families.

A business decision determines how best to make a business service or product more attractive to consumers. In contrast, there is no need to make a necessary healthcare service more attractive to the consumer (patient). The consumer (patient) must have the service.

A business decision determines how best to have a business service generate a profit in order for the business to remain in business. In contrast, a healthcare decision determines how best to have a healthcare service maintain and restore health. Remaining in business is not a problem for the healthcare industry.

Both the quality and the availability of a business service or product can be modified, but neither the quality nor the availability of a necessary healthcare service or product can be modified.

Increasing the cost of a business service may discourage its purchase. Increasing the cost of a healthcare service will not discourage its purchase. Patients must have the service.

Business services can be restrict to only those consumers who can afford to purchase them, and the charges for those services can be adjusted to whatever the consumer is willing to pay. However, healthcare services can not be restricted to only those consumers (patients) who can afford to purchase them, and since patients must have the services, the charges for those services can not be adjusted to whatever the consumer (patient) is willing to pay. Furthermore, since the patient is no longer responsible for paying for their services (insurance pays), price controls have become necessary.

Discussing the differences between business and heathcare is not intended to be critical of the business community. A strong and profitable business community is essential to maintaining a private healthcare delivery system. The discussion amplifies only why the healthcare delivery system is different than a business system, and it explains why healthcare can not be managed successfully as a business. If one wishes to apply the word "manage" to healthcare, healthcare's costs and its service utilization are best managed by physicians using the proposed six changes to regulate a private healthcare delivery system.

The unsuccessful management of healthcare as a business system introduces the next topic—HMOs, Patients Beware!

Addendum III

The HMO
Patients Beware!

HMO is the acronym for Hand the Money Over.

Yes, HMOs are removing billions of dollars from the healthcare delivery system:

1. to pay investors their dividends.

2. to pay generous management salaries and benefits.

3. to pay expensive marketing and advertising costs, and

4. to pay other administrative and operating expenses.

Those billions of dollars would be better spent purchasing healthcare services in a private healthcare delivery system whose service costs and service utilization are regulated by the recommended six changes.

What is an HMO?

An HMO is neither an insurance company nor a provider. It is a business! It buys and sells healthcare services for a profit. It contracts with a variety of healthcare providers to buy their services at a specified price, and it manages the sale (distribution) of those services by controlling when, where, and from whom the HMO's enrollees receive those services.

In contrast, a private indemnity insurance company is not a business. It neither buys nor sells healthcare services. Instead, it is a broker. It transfers the money it receives from its policyholder's premiums to the providers who have offered those policyholders services, and it does not control when, where, or from whom its policyholders receive their services.

A question frequently asked is how can an HMO offer a less expensive premium than an indemnity insurance company? Isn't this an example of an HMO's ability to save healthcare dollars? No! No!! No!!!

HMOs have been able to offer less expensive premiums because:

1. they have been able to restrict their enrollments to the 80% of the population who have no disabilities or chronic illnesses,

2. they have been able to deny their enrollees services,

3. they have been able to control the amount of the reimbursements they offer their providers,

4. they have been able to control when, where, and from whom their enrolles receive their services, and

5. they have had immunity from lawsuits.

In contrast, a private indemnity insurance company has more expensive premiums because:

1. they enroll everyone, including individuals with preexisting disabilities and chronic illnesses,

2. they do not deny their policyholders any services,

3. they do not control their provider's reimbursements, and

4. they do not control when, where, and from whom their policyholders receive their services.

An HMO's immunity from lawsuits, its ability to restrict its enrollments to individuals with no disabilities or chronic illnesses, and its ability to control its provider's reinbursements has offered HMOs a significant cost advantage over competing private indemnity insurance companies.

For example, individuals with disabilities and chronic illnessess create an estimated 65% of healthcare's costs. Since indemnity insurance companies accept these individuals and HMOs do not accept them, the cost of the services offered to indemnity insurance company's policyholders are 65% more expensive than the cost of the services offered to HMO enrollees. Or, HMOs can anticipate saving 65% of an indemnity insurance company's service costs.

If the cost of the services an indemnity insurance company offers its policyholders requires a $6,000 premium, 65% of those service costs have been generated by their policyholders with disabilities and chronic illnesses. 65% of the insurance company's $6,000 premium is $3,900. The remaining $2,100 of the $6,000 premium pays for the services the company provides its policyholders with no disabilities or chronic illnesses.

Since the HMO has been able to avoid enrolling individuals with disabilities and chronic illnesses, the HMO can anticipate having to spend only the $2,100 the indemnity insurance company spends for its services to its policyholders with no disabilities or chronic illnesses. The HMO does not have to spend the $3,900 the indemnity insurance company had to spend to offer services to its policyholders with disabilities and chronic illnesses. If the cost of an HMOs premium is only $5,000, after spending the $2,100 for its enrollees's services, the HMO has $2,900 remaining from its $5,000 premium. Or, the HMO obtained a generous profit of $2,900. Due to their selective enrollment policies, the HMO was able to obtain a $2,900 profit from its $5,000 premium while the indemnity insurance company was able to obtain no profit from its $6,000 premium. Have you believed HMOs were there to benefit the public?

Those less expensive HMO premiums have caused a serious problem for the indemnity insurance industry. The less expensive HMO premiums have attracted an increasing number of the 80% of the population who have no disabilities or chronic illnesses. Their less expensive service costs had offered the indemnity insurance industry the opportunity to apply some of their premiums towards the costs of the more expensive services required by their policyholders with disabilities and chronic illnesses. The loss of those less expensive policyholders to the HMOs, and their need to continue to offer the more expensive services to their policyholders with disabilities and chronic illnesses has increased the cost of the indemnity insurance industry's premiums. Over the past two decades, those premiums have become prohibitively expensive.

These prohibitively expensive premiums are forcing the collapse of the private health insurance industry. Congress created the HMO industry to compete with, and ultimately destroy, the private insurance industry, and Congress has been successful.

The Future of HMOs.

The future of the HMO industry depends on Congress. The industry can be easily destroyed by two legislative mandates. One is to require HMOs to enroll everyone who applies, regardless of preexisting disabilities or chronic illnesses, and the other is to allow HMOs to be sued. (The "Patient's Bill of Rights" legislation.)

If the HMO industry were required to enroll everyone, the added cost of providing services to enrollees with disabilities and chronic illnesses would increase their service costs significantly. If those increased service costs were added to an HMO's existing investor, management, marketing, advertising, and other administrative costs, the HMO's operating costs would become greater than those of the competing private indemnity insurance industry. Those more expensive operating costs would force the HMO's premiums to become more expensive than those offered by the private indemnity insurance industry, and:

1. HMOs would be less attractive to the public.

2. HMO enrollments would decline.

3. The ability of HMOs to generate profits and support its management and administrative infrastructure would become difficult.

4. Both enrollees and investors would abandon the HMO industry, and

5. the HMO industry would become bankrupt and collapse.

The second option Congress has to destroy the HMO industry is to expose it to lawsuits. The cost of defending themselves from a flood of enrollee initiated lawsuits would drive the HMOs into bankruptcy (the "Patient's Bill of Rights" legislation). However, bankruptcy would not be the end of the HMO industry. The industry's existing infrastructure would be absorbed by government to become the management and delivery system for their National Health Service.

Would a union of the HMO industry with a government sponsored National Health Service benefit the public? The answer is no, and the reasons have been discussed. However, the public may have to make a decision within this decade of whether or not the private delivery system is worth preserving. Will the public allow government to replace the private healthcare delivery system with a National Health Service whose services are offered by the HMO industry?

History as shown the centralization of power is always associated with the abuse of that power, and both the HMO industry and government are examples. Over the past three decades, increasing HMO enrollments have offered the HMO industry increasing power, and as their power increased, they became more arrogant and less provider and less patient friendly.

Based on my expriences as the Medical Director of an HMO, HMO's management thinks of physicians as only the suppliers of their services. They fail to recognize the quality of the HMO's services depends on the quality of their physicians. Furthermore, they believe physcians should be their employees rather than independent contractors. In addition, HMO's management believes enrollees are numbers who generate costs rather than patients requiring treatment for their diseases and disorders, and they believe their enrollee's services are negotiable commodities.

Likewise, the centralization of power within government is always associated with the creation of expensive bureaucracies and the suppliers of inferior services. The Department of Education is an example.

Hopefully, the profit driven HMO industry will never be given the opportunity to become the delivery system for the public's healthcare services.

Epilogue

My journey into medicine began in 1949. Prior to me, there had been two generations of physicians in my family, and becoming a physician had been my wish since childhood. But in 2003, I find myself asking the question: What does the future hold for medicine?

Unfortuately, during the three decades prior to 2003, neither patients nor physicians have been thinking beyond their tomorrow. Physicians are benefiting from the large incomes insurance is providing them, and patients are benefiting from the free services insurance is providing them. However, in the next decade, much to their surprise, they will discover those insurance programs have been neither a benefit nor without cost.

Yes, at my age, I will probably not have the opportunity to witness medicine in 2013. But, lets look at what I beleive medicine could be in 2013. Many individuals are unhappy over the loss of the many benefits they remember having received from the private healthcare delivery system. A National Health Service has replaced the private healthcare delivery system, and the public has been assigned a managed healthcare company (HMO) to offer them their medical, surgical, and hospital services. Many individuals are dissatisfied with both the attitude of, and the services provided by, the physicians employed by their managed healthcare company (HMO). In contrast, both the government and the HMO industry are content. The public's dependency on government for their medical and surgical services has provided government the power they were seeking, and the investors in the HMO industry are obtaining the profits they were seeking.

But, what about the unhappy public? Who? Oh yes, them. They were offered the opportunity to control healthcare a decade ago, but they did nothing. Now, it is too late. Too bad!

What about physicians? The loss of the private healthcare delivery system has forced them to become salaried employees in managed healthcare companies. Too bad!

The loss of the private healthcare delivery system was caused by the failure of the public to think beyond tomorrow back in 2003. An example is how foolish the public was in 2003 to continue harrassing their employers with strikes demanding increased healthcare benefits to pay for their increasing healthcare costs. If they had thought about the long range consequences of increasing healthcare costs, instead of striking, they would have joined with their employers to reduce healthcare's costs. Reducing those costs would have preserved the private healthcare delivery system and would have encouraged employers to retain their businesses in the United States. In 2003, employers were paying the highest business taxes, the most expensive employee healthcare benefits, and the most expensive litigation costs in the industrialized world. Is there any question why many employers have taken their manufacturing businesses and jobs out of the United States.

Perhaps the most significant problem for the public in 2013 is their physicians. The public's primary care physicians are nine-to-five salaried employees of HMOs, and referrals to specialists are increasingly more difficult to obtain. Also, since physicians have become salaried employees of managed healthcare companies, the applications to Medical Schools have declined significantly as has the academic credentials of those applying. A person with the academic ability to choose any career of their choice is not considering healthcare as a career.

To avoid what I have just described as what I believe medicine will be in 2013, the public is encouraged to support the six changes discussed in this book to regulate a private healthcare delivery system. The six changes will reduce healthcare's costs by 25% to 30% within two years and as much as 40% within five years; will reduce litigation costs by about 70%; will provide everyone unable to pay for their services the opportuity to obtain quality and easily available services in free healthcare facilities; and will provide the careeer incentives necessary to attract the best from among our youth into healthcare to become the physicians of the future.

After reading this book, the public needs to ponder the following questions.

Is a private healthcare delivery system important to me and to my family?

Are physicians important to the quality and availability of the public's healthcare services?

Does a private healthcare delivery system offer the best opportunity to attract the best from among our youth into healthcare to become the future physicians?

Hopefully, the public's answer to all is yes, and they will become the healthcare activists required to preserve the private healthcare delivery system.

0-595-29213-5